INSIGHTS
of a
SENIOR
ACUPUNCTURIST

BY
MIRIAM LEE
BLUE POPPY PRESS

Published by:
BLUE POPPY PRESS
A Division of Blue Poppy Enterprises, Inc.
1990 N 57th Court, Unit A
BOULDER, CO 80301

First Edition, February, 1992
Second Printing, December, 1993
Third Edition, March, 1994
Fourth Printing, February, 1996
Fifth Printing, February, 1998
Sixth Printing, May, 1999
Seventh Printing, April, 2001
Eighth Printing, March, 2003
Ninth Printing, August, 2004
Tenth Printing, April, 2006
Eleventh Printing, March, 2007
Twelfth Printing, December, 2007
Thirteenth Printing, December, 2008
Fourteenth Printing, November, 2009
Fifteenth Printing, May, 2010
Sixteenth Printing, September, 2011
Seventeenth Printing, June, 2012
Eighteenth Printing, January, 2013

ISBN 0-936185-33-3   ISBN 978-0-936185-33-0

DISCLAIMER: The information in this book is given in good faith. However, the author and the publishers cannot be held responsible for any error or omission. The publishers will not accept liabilities for any injuries or damages caused to the reader that may result from the reader's acting upon or using the content contained in this book. The publishers make this information available to English language readers for research and scholarly purposes only.

The publishers do not advocate nor endorse self-medication by laypersons. Chinese medicine is a professional medicine. Laypersons interested in availing themselves of the treatments described in this book should seek out a qualified professional practitioner of Chinese medicine.

COMP Designation: Original work

20 19 18

Printed at Edwards Brothers Malloy, Ann Arbor, MI
Cover design by Anne Rue

Foreword

In the Autumn of 1991 Blue Poppy Press did a survey of our buyers requesting information about what types of books they felt they needed in order to be more effective practitioners. While the answers were many and varied, the overwhelming majority of respondents mentioned a need for more books on acupuncture treatment, and specifically books which would present alternatives to or at least expand upon the TCM acupuncture that most American practitioners have learned in acupuncture schools both here and/or in China. This book is an initial, and we hope well received, response to these requests.

Miriam Lee, OMD, is an acupuncturist of prodigious skill and well deserved fame in her home state of California. She has honed the art and science of acupuncture for over 40 years, and, while there may be many "old masters" or senior practitioners now living and working in the U.S., very few of them have chosen to share their knowledge through writing or teaching as Miriam has. She has taught hundreds of students both privately and as a lecturer at schools and colleges of acupuncture. Additionally, she has been a powerful force for acupuncture in the legislative process in California, and she has treated literally thousands of patients.

Miriam was trained as an acupuncturist in China prior to "Liberation" in 1949. Her training therefore, was prior to the ascendance of the style of acupuncture which has come to be called Traditional Chinese Medicine (TCM), the style in which most acupuncturists in the United States and almost all acupuncturists in the People's Republic of China are currently trained. The fact that TCM acupuncture is, in fact, only one style of acupuncture has been well documented by several writers in recent years[1].

---

[1]   Hammer, Leon I., "Dueling Needles: Reflections on the Politics of Medical Models", *American Journal of Acupuncture (AJA)*, USA, Vol. 19, #3, 1991

A discussion of the merits or drawbacks of this style could fill an entire book and I will not belabor that question here. Suffice it to say that while a great deal has been written on the practice of TCM acupuncture, other styles from Japan, Korea, Vietnam, or pre-TCM Chinese lineages are only recently being explored by most American acupuncturists as viable, clinically effective alternatives. As publishers it is our desire to encourage this exploration.

Moreover, since we are practitioners as well as publishers, we have several other reasons for wanting to make available this useful book by Miriam Lee. We have used the treatments and the ideas that Miriam discusses here in our own clinical work and we found that, not only were her treatments effective, they encouraged us as acupuncturists to explore and expand our ideas about our art. While the main treatment protocol discussed herein can be safely and effectively used by beginning acupuncturists, it is also subtle enough in its application of acupuncture theory to be appreciated by even the most advanced practitioner. And, as I personally have had the good fortune to spend a short time observing at Miriam's clinic in Palo Alto, I have seen the effectiveness of her use of this protocol first hand.

Perhaps the most interesting aspect of this book is the deceptive simplicity of the main protocol described. While using only 5 very commonplace acupoints, *Zu San Li* (St 36), *San Yin Jiao* (Sp 6), *He Gu* (LI 4), *Qu Chi* (LI 11), and *Lie Que* (Lu 7), as the basis for treating a wide variety of ills, much of the theoretical material supporting their use is both profound and somewhat unorthodox in the sense that it is definitely not what is taught in any TCM textbooks translated into English to date. Miriam's writing style is conversational and easy to read and understand, but her perspective on point selection and usage, channel and *zang fu* theory, needle technique, and on how and why to practice acupuncture offer all practitioners fresh food for thought. She is able to express her own continued respect and awe for the art that she practices so well. She is able to help us remember the magical aspect of practicing acupuncture, the reason that so many of us were drawn

---

Flaws, Bob, *Before Completion Essays on the Practice of TCM*, Blue Poppy Press, Boulder, CO, Feb., 1992

to study it in the first place. We at Blue Poppy Press hope that this book may help in a small way to bring the work of this notable practitioner to a larger audience.

Honora Lee Wolfe
January 28, 1992

Collaborator's Preface

In the classical acupuncture literature of China there are many references to specific point combinations used by famous physicians. These point combinations have such a powerful therapeutic effect that they have been passed on and used throughout history. Once recognized as belonging to this category, powerful formulas were then included in the medical literature.

Miriam Lee has formulated such a combination of points and its use has been refined into an art in her clinic. In this book she shares her knowledge of the point formula: *Zu San Li* (St 36), *San Yin Jiao* (Sp 6), *He Gu* (LI 4), *Qu Chi* (LI 11), and *Lie Que* (Lu 7).

As her student for the last 3 years, I have seen her obtain excellent results with this formula. In helping her to write this book, I have come to understand in a much deeper way why it is that her treatments work so well. Her careful explanation of technique and intention has enabled me, as a beginning acupuncturist, to better utilize the energy of the points and channels when treating my own patients.

Lela Carney

Author's Preface

I came to the United States from Singapore where I had lived for 17 years after leaving mainland China in 1949. In China I had been a nurse and a midwife before becoming an acupuncturist, and I had lived through the Japanese occupation and World War II, extremely difficult times in a land accustomed to hard times.

Life is easier in Singapore than it is in China, and as an acupuncturist, I began seeing there the kinds of problems that arise from unfairness and anger which are so common in America. Treatments for depression, hyperactivity, and mental problems such as schizophrenia or suicide are not discussed in acupuncture books from China. There the struggle for life itself takes so much energy that few people are able to suffer anguish over the *quality* of life. In Singapore as in America, there is enough bread, and so there is more qi caught up in emotional blockages.

When I first came to California acupuncture was illegal. I worked on an assembly line at Hewlett Packard and attended church, building a life for myself in this country where my medicine was against the law. I could only wait to see how I would be called upon to give what I had learned.

A young Chinese man with a PhD from Stanford was the son of a member of my church. He had had a tumor removed from the *ming men* area of his spine, and after the operation he could not walk. I told his mother that acupuncture could help, and went to him every other day. With treatment he began to walk and was able to get a job.

The mother then sent me an American lady in her 50's. She worked in a restaurant and could not raise her arm to carry the trays. After one treatment she was free of pain. She sent a friend who worked for *Sunset* magazine. This woman had had low back pain for six years and the doctors recommended surgery. She refused to let them operate, but was reduced to working one hour a day. She was quite a large lady, and I had not prepared long enough needles. Nevertheless, I treated her with a prayerful heart.

After three days she stood outside my house shouting. I was scared, but I cautiously opened the door to see what was going on. She told me she had gone home after the treatment and had scrubbed every corner of her house. She had cleaned for 17 hours, and her back did not hurt. She sent me everyone in her office.

Many people began to come for treatments. Because acupuncture was still illegal, no one would rent me an office, and people came to my house. They came up the back staircase, and at one point there were so many people waiting on the stairs to get in the staircase broke.

In 1973 Dr. Harry Oxenhandler, an M.D., offered to share his office with me. I could only practice for a limited amount of time each day, until 1 P.M. I had to start earlier and earlier in the morning. By 5 A.M. there were 4 or 5 people waiting in their cars to get in. So for 7 hours a day, 5 days a week, I saw between 75 and 80 patients a day, 14 to 17 patients an hour. I had 4 beds for those who had to lie down. People in wheelchairs were treated in the bathroom. Those who could sit I treated in the waiting room or on the foot of the treatment tables. I worked alone, putting in and taking out the needles, and recording all the treatments. The pressure was tremendous. I had to come up with a safe, effective treatment that I could apply quickly and easily to people with ordinary sicknesses so that I could focus on those with really difficult conditions.

There is an old Chinese saying, "If you don't press the olive seed, there will be no oil." The pressure was a great challenge for me. In the afternoons and evenings I poured over the classics looking for guidance. In the *Nei Jing* I found my starting point:

> When the stomach and spleen, the central *jiao*, are attacked by emotion, pure qi cannot ascend to the brain, and the evil qi, the waste, cannot descend. It will remain stuck in the stomach.

In the Western way of thinking pure qi is oxygen; the evil qi, or waste, is carbon dioxide. When there is no pure qi or oxygen in the head, the person thinks only on the darker side, and death seems like the only possible solution to life's difficulties.

Zu San Li (St 36) is the best point to free stuck qi in the central *jiao*. You can drain or supplement it to make the pure qi go up. Because many cases of depression are due to stagnant liver qi, I chose *San Yin Jiao* (Sp 6) to help the liver along with the kidneys and spleen.

I also needed a way to make the evil qi go down, to drain it. Draining *Qu Chi* (LI 11) and *He Gu* (LI 4) drains evil qi from the body. *Qu Chi* (LI 11) helps move the bowel, clearing waste from the intestines. Draining *Lie Que* (Lu 7) clears the kidneys as well, and the kidneys rule the brain. When the brain has enough oxygen, then the person thinks on the brighter side again.

Because the stomach and large intestine channels have more qi and more blood, you can do no harm by treating them at any time for any person. These 10 needles have allowed me to think fast, treat fast. They are safe for new hands, and can be used successfully by those who do not yet know how to diagnose. They served me well during those years when I had no time for diagnosis beyond recognizing "here is a person whose central *jiao* has been attacked by emotion".

On April 15, 1974, Governor Reagan vetoed a bill legalizing the practice of acupuncture in California. I was arrested for practicing medicine without a license on April 16. The police came at 6:45 A.M. when I already had 10 people in the office. I had to take the needles out and let them go. Some had driven a long way to be treated, including one from Redding, 4 hours away.

At the trial my patients filled the courtroom. There were so many of them court officials didn't know what to do with them all. Day after day they returned to protest being denied access to the only medicine which had helped them, and to insist that they had a right to choose to be treated with acupuncture. Within a matter of days legislators reached a compromise with Governor Reagan, and acupuncture was made an "experimental procedure" which could be carried out as research. I was made part of a project at San Francisco University and practiced under this umbrella until Governor Jerry Brown signed the legislation legalizing acupuncture in 1976.

As I said, this 10 needle treatment is safe for new hands. I have students who told me they have applied these points for 6 years, and the treatments have never failed. When they record these treatments they simple write "M.L. Great", for "Miriam Lee's Great 10 Needle Treatment".

Contents

Section 1: Theoretical Models

Section 2: The Clinical Applications of *Zu San Li* (St 36), *San Yin Jiao* (Sp 6), *He Gu* (LI 4), *Qu Chi* (LI 11), & *Lie Que* (Lu 7): One Combination of Points Can Treat Many Diseases

Appendices

Section 1
Theoretical Models

1

Antique Points

The points which are most commonly used in acupuncture treatment are located at or below the knee and elbow. These points, collectively known as the antique points, include the five phase points, *yuan* source, *luo* connecting, and *xi* cleft points, the lower *he* sea points, and the *hui* reunion points of the eight extraordinary vessels.

Treating these antique points gives good results for local, channel, and internal organ diseases, and for this reason they are used by the most advanced practitioners as well as being the first points taught to beginning students. To master the use of even a few of these points gives the practitioner command over many diseases. In my own practice, I have formulated a combination of these points which gives exceptional results: *Zu San Li* (St 36), *San Yin Jiao* (Sp 6), *He Gu* (LI 4), *Qu Chi* (LI 11), and *Lie Que* (Lu 7).

Why, we may wonder, do points so far away from the crucial organs and control centers of the body have such a profound effect? Research has been done in China to determine the nature, in Western physiological terms, of the body's response to stimulation of these points.

Nerve endings in the extremities are very sensitive. They are near the ends of their pathways from the brain for motor nerves or near the beginning of the pathways to the brain for sensory nerves. The reflex action to the subcortex is very strong when points on the extremities are stimulated. Whereas, the reflex action to the brain is smaller when stimulation is applied at the location of pain or disease itself. Research has shown that the further away from the brain and/or from the site of the problem stimulation is given, the stronger the reflex will be. This is especially so when the site of stimulation is on the extremities and at one of the points classically recognized as an antique point.

The hands and feet are the most physically active part of the body. They move the most. The hands to work and the feet to carry the body from one place to another. Therefore, they have more energy flowing through them available for the acupuncturist to tap. This, of course, is an explanation in keeping with traditional Chinese physiology which emphasizes function and energy in its qualitative aspects rather than structure and the quantitative measurement of processes so important to Western science.

In traditional Chinese anatomy, the energies of the yin channels of the hand and the yang channels of the leg are at their most yin and yang respectively as they reach their ends at the tips of the fingers and toes. Points at the ends of these channels are also the most unstable or radical in their action since these are the pivot points where the energy of one channel changes to the opposite polarity of the channel which follows it. For instance, yin energy of the hand *tai yin* lung changes to the yang energy of the hand *yang ming* large intestine, hand *jue yin* pericardium to hand *shao yang* triple heater, hand *shao yin* heart to hand *tai yang* small intestine. The yang channels of the hand and the yin channels of the leg which also begin at the extremities are unstable in energy and strong in action in the same way. Yang changes to yin as the qi of the foot *yang ming* flows into the foot *tai yin*, foot *shao yang* to foot *jue yin*, foot *tai yang* to foot *shao yin*.

An example of the strength of the energy at the ends of the extremities is the use of the *Shi Xuan* or Ten Spreadings (M-UE-49), for yang windstroke or apoplexy of the full type. These points at the tips of the 10 fingers are bled to drain fullness, thereby allowing the red flush to drain from the face, the eyes and mouth to close, the hands to unclench, the coarse breathing to calm, and consciousness to return to the patient. The 10 *jing* well points can also be bled for this purpose, but the tips of the fingers are easier to get to and thus easier to use on patients in such an extreme condition.

4

A. Points Near the Thumb & Great Toe

The action of points on both the thumb and the great toe are different from that of points on the other fingers and toes. In studies of the physiological response of the brain to acupuncture, these points have demonstrated a more powerful reflex to the subcortex than other distal points. Western hand and foot reflexology also recognizes the effect points on the thumb and great toe have on diseases of the head and dysfunction of the master regulatory endocrine glands located in the head.

He Gu (LI 4) and *Tai Chong* (Liv 3) are near the thumb and great toe respectively, as well as being the *yuan* source points of their respective channels. Their use is a prime example of the power of points in these locations. Needling them together is called "opening the Four Gates". This treatment is used for complicated cases in which yin and yang symptoms are mixed, such as mental disturbance and drug addiction.[2]

B. Five Phase Points

From the ends of the fingers and toes upward, the order of progression of the points, according to the five phases is as follows: in yin channels, the first point corresponds to wood. Then, according to the *sheng* or generation cycle come fire, earth, metal, and water, all water points on the yin channels being located at the elbows and knees. In yang channels, the first point corresponds to metal. Then according to the generation cycle come water, wood, fire, and earth, all earth points on yang channels being located at the elbows and knees.

One should note that there is a relationship between the pairs of points as they progress up the extremities as well. The first points are metal and wood on the yang and yin channels respectively. Then come water and fire, wood and earth, fire and metal, earth and water. This is according to the control or *ke* cycle of the five phases, and has to do with the special relationship of

---

[2]   Their use is more appropriate in cases of fullness, liver qi congestion, and emotional imbalance in strong patients than in weak patients with empty signs and symptoms.

yin and yang in Chinese medicine. The control cycle is not an antagonistic process in the healthy person but a beneficial one. The paired phases keep each other's activities with appropriate bounds just as a soft and tender-hearted woman can manage a wild, unruly husband. Under loving control, he can work and provide for his family.

Chinese theory often makes use of family relationships as descriptive metaphors. There is the relationship of wife to husband which is used to describe the paired yin and yang organs and channels. There is the mother-son relationship which is used when describing the *sheng* cycle. And there is the grandmother-grandson relationship used to describe the *ke* cycle. Though husband and wife are different, together they function harmoniously. Parents nourish their children, and grandparents show them their place in the scheme of things.

C. The Transport Points

From a five phase point of view, the first points on the extremities correspond to different phases as do the second, third, fourth, and fifth. As such, each has different functions and applications. However, points in the same location or order in the sequence also have certain actions in common. These common functions are based on another system of categorizing these points. When referred to from this other point of view, these same points are called the *wu shu xue* or 5 transport points. According to this system each of these 5 points from fingers to elbows and from toes to knees is identified from distal to proximal as either *jing* well, *rong* gushing, *shu* transporting, *jing* traversing, or *he* uniting points. Because they represent the growth or increasing strength of qi in the channels as it moves from the ends of the extremities up to the elbow and knee joints, another translation or interpretation calls these same points the well, spring, stream, river, and sea points. Both sets of terms are useful to give an image of the quality of qi which is available in these points as will be seen from the following explanation of each type of point. In this system, both yin and yang points on the same level are categorized the same and are given the same name, *e.g.*, *jing, rong, shu, jing,* or *he.* (See Appendix A.)

The first point is the *jing* well point. Its energy is like water being drawn from a well. You remove one bucketful and more water comes to replace it. The level does not rise or fall and it never overflows, but it must be drawn from. In treatment, well points are most often pricked and squeezed for bleeding.

The second point is the *rong* spring point. Water gushes from the spring on its own. Unlike the well, it does not have to be pumped or drawn. Its flow is shallow and small.

The third point is the *shu* stream point. It is substantial and has a definite direction. It also has more qi than the two previous points.

The *jing* river point is stronger and broader yet and can carry more.

Finally, in the *he* sea points, the qi spreads and unites with the body's qi as a whole as rivers merge into the sea. The qi here is great and deep. The *he* sea points tap the body's most extensive energetic resources and regulate its overall functioning.

According to the *Ling Shu*, the 5 transport points are used as follows: the *jing* well points are used to treat diseases of the *zang* organs. If there are changes in color, *rong* spring points are used. For chronic conditions use the *shu* stream points. For conditions in which the voice changes, use *jing* river points. And *he* sea points are for problems due to irregular eating.

To be clinically useful, these categories must be further explained. *Jing* well point are used for acute infections, sudden severe pain, and sudden changes in emotion. One example is a sudden sore throat with swelling and difficulty swallowing, due to eating too much hot, spicy food. In this instance, the *zang* and *fu* organs' activities are imbalanced and heat goes up when it should be going down. To treat this condition, bleed *Shang Yang* (LI 1), and *Shao Shang* (Lu 11) to clear heat (*qing re*) from the lung, large intestine, and stomach organs. When there is phlegm accumulation in the channels and orifices, not in the lungs, the qi cannot flow freely. This can lead to stroke, madness, and, in the case of fever or extreme environmental heat, convulsion or heat stroke. Bleeding the 10 *jing* well points or *Shi Xuan* (M-UE-49) as mentioned above is the appropriate treatment to drain fullness (*xie shi*) and open the channels (*tong jing*).

7

Using the spleen channel's *jing* well point together with the stomach *jing* well point calms the spirit so that the patient can sleep without nightmares. *Tai Bai* (Sp 1) with *Da Dun* (Liv 1) treats hemorrhage because the spleen controls the blood and the liver stores blood. In treating hemorrhage, these points are moxaed because the condition is one of emptiness. Bleeding is for draining full conditions.

Bleeding the heart and small intestine *jing* well points, *Shao Chong* (Ht 9) and *Shao Ze* (SI 1) clears heat and tranquilizes the heart. This combination is used for sudden stroke where the patient falls unconscious and is breathing hard with phlegm gurgling in the throat. In this case, the face turns purple. This distinguishes it from other phlegm obstruction situations where all 10 well points or the *Shi Xuan* (M-UE-49) are used.

Moxa at *Zhi Yin* (Bl 67) adjusts the position of the fetus and helps ease difficult childbirth. *Yong Quan* (Ki 1) is used to treat energy which is flowing the wrong way, as in infantile convulsions with high fever, convulsions due to sudden fright or shock, and epilepsy. This use of the point relates to its being the wood point on the bottom of the foot. When liver wind goes to the top of the head, as in seizures or convulsions, *Yong Quan* (Ki 1) is useful in controlling this and bringing it back down.[3] Needle it with strong stimulation; do not moxa.

Moxa on *Zhong Chong* (Per 9) and *Guan Chong* (TH 1) is used to treat people who suddenly lose yang. This is a condition of cold collapse and is another form of stroke. The face in this instance is pale, the eyes are closed, and there is profuse cold perspiration.

Needle *Zu Qiao Yin* (GB 44) for insomnia.

The above conditions are all considered to be diseases which originate in the organs and not in the channels themselves. They are generally acute, severe, emergency conditions.

---

[3]   Wind is related to wood in the five phases.

Sudden changes in emotion which cause the face to become pale or flushed are also treated with the *jing* well points and not *rong* spring points. *Rong* spring points are only used when the beginning stages of a disease causes a change in facial color. For example, in acute bronchitis or pneumonia, heat in the lungs causes the cheeks to be red in the beginning. Draining *Yu Ji* (Lu 10) and *Er Jian* (LI 2) clears the heat and disinhibits the bronchi, thus making breathing less difficult.

When the patient fears acupuncture or begins to faint after needles are inserted, their face becomes pale. *Shao Fu* (Ht 8) is drained to revive them. In this case, stimulation of *xie fa* or draining technique actually revives. If, on the other hand, fingers are closed after a stroke, supplement *Shao Fu* (Ht 8). There is also a kind of nerve pain which is relieved by *rong* spring points. If evil qi counterflows laterally (*heng ni*) into the flanks causing pain, draining *Xing Jian* (Liv 2) will induce the liver qi to descend, thus eliminating pain and congestion from the sides.

Ye Men (TH 2) and *Yu Ji* (Lu 10) are used together with *xie fa* or draining technique in classical formulas to stop the pain of sore throat. But in my clinical experience *Yu Ji* (Lu 10) is a very painful point to needle, no matter how good the acupuncturist's technique. Therefore, I use *Chi Ze* (Lu 5) instead. *Yu Ji* (Lu 10) is also indicated for cold pain in the Stomach.

Shu stream points, which on yin channels are also the *yuan* source points, are used for chronic conditions which come and go. This includes any kind of intermittent fever or pain, such as nerve pain, headache, arthritis which is fine in good weather but returns in rainy, windy, cold weather, malaria, epilepsy, and occasional recurring shooting pains. Examples in relation to headaches include the use of *Shu Gu* (Bl 65) for pain at the top of the head, *Xian Gu* (St 43) for frontal headache, and *Zu Ling Qi* (GB 41) for one-sided migrainous headaches.

Jing river points are used not only for voice changes but any speech difficulty resulting from loss of balance in the organs. *Jing Gu* (Lu 8) is used for any kind of cough, but especially for that which sounds like a broken gong. It has no resonance, but sounds jagged and flat. This kind of cough often appears in pneumonia. While *Jing Gu* (Lu 8) adjusts the respiratory system, it is located near the radial artery. Though theory calls for it use, *Chi Ze* (Lu 5) is safer clinically. Thus it can be seen that point selection must always be made taking a number of factors into account: theory, knowledge of specific point functions, the safety of points, *i.e.*, their anatomical location near organs or blood vessels, and how painful they are to needle. While the theories are valuable, they must be used flexibly.

Ling Dao (Ht 4) is for sudden loss of voice and cough due to heart channel imbalance. This treatment uses the metal point on the fire channel to treat the lungs.

Yang Gu (SI 5) is for swollen jaw and inability to open the jaw, *i.e.*, lockjaw.

Jian Shi (Per 5) is for loss of voice due to heart heat or cold, or heat and cold mixed (fire against metal again) and inability to open the mouth.

Fu Liu (Ki 7) is for wheezing as is *Kun Lun* (Bl 60). *Kun Lun* (Bl 60) can also be used for toothache.

Yang Xi (LI 5) treats sore throat and hoarseness, but *Jie Xi* (St 41) treats bloodshot eyes and edema of the face, the kind caused by fluid retention. In other words, not all uses of the points conform to transport system theory. Some can be seen to relate more to their five phase functions.

He sea points adjust and balance the physiological activity of the inner organs, especially when the problem is due to irregular eating. For digestive diseases, *Zu San Li* (St. 36), *Yin Ling Quan* (Sp 9), and *Qu Chi* (LI 11) in combination increase the power of digestion, metabolism, and respiration. Their use strengthens the body and increases health.

The most powerful of the *he* sea points, *Zu San Li* (St 36), adjusts the qi and blood of all the channels and strengthens the spleen and stomach. It is one of the major supplementation points of the body and has the ability to treat a broad range of conditions. It tranquilizes the spirit and, when used frequently, increases health and vitality. Because it supplements the kidney, it increases the power of seeing and hearing.

Current research has found that *Zu San Li* (St 36) can both increase and decrease the motility of the stomach. It can both raise and lower blood pressure, and its use increases or decreases the white blood cell count depending upon whether there are already too few or too many white blood cells. This regulatory function makes *Zu San Li* (St 36) useful in many seemingly different and contradictory conditions.

After overeating, food may stagnate in the stomach. No qi, food, or gas can pass through. The abdomen becomes bloated and pain results. Or, if one becomes angry after eating, digestion stops and food stays in the stomach. Stimulation of *Zu San Li* (St 36) both increases the secretion of hydrochloric acid and regulates the circulation of qi, dissolving food and moving it out of the stomach. Because it increases the acid in the stomach, *Zu San Li* (St 36) is not used for ulcers.

For cases of emaciation, it can be supplemented to restore appetite and strength. Use moxa in addition to needles for very weak patients. For acute, severe stomach pain, bleed *Zu San Li* (St 36) with a triangle needle and the symptoms will disappear.

The *he* sea or uniting point of the large intestine, *Qu Chi* (LI 11) is used to treat diseases of the *fu* bowels or hollow organ diseases. It dispels wind and relieves the surface. It also regulates the qi. Current research in China has found that stimulating *Qu Chi* (LI 11) increases white blood cells, thus increasing immune competence and providing an anti-biotic, anti-inflammatory action.

D. *Yuan* Source & *Luo* Connecting Points

Yuan source and *luo* connecting points of paired yin and yang channels/organs are used in combination to take advantage of the relationship between the two. *He Gu* (LI 4) and *Lie Que* (Lu 7) are an especially powerful pair of *yuan* source and *luo* connecting points. The *yuan* source point of the large intestine channel, *He Gu* (LI 4), can open both the large intestine and the lungs and thus treats lung related diseases.

He Gu (LI 4) is one of the thumb points which have special influence on the brain. It is used to treat many kinds of diseases, especially those from the neck up. Special areas of action are the teeth, jaws, and throat through which the large intestine channel passes before its termination at the nose.

Luo points have a number of special characteristics. Yin *luo* points draw on the qi of their paired yang channel. Yang *luo* points draw on the yang channel qi also. You cannot tap the yin through the *luo* points. In addition, the qi of yang channels flows in both directions, forward and backward, simultaneously. The qi in yin channels goes in only one direction and does not return until the next 24 hour cycle. Thus the *luo* point connecting the yin channel to the yang channel taps qi which is always coming and going. Because of this, the *luo* points of the yin channels can be used at any time.

Lie Que (Lu 7), like *He Gu* (LI 4), takes care of all trouble of the head and neck. It can also be used for diagnosis. It is swollen, big and puffy, the disease is one of fullness (*shi*), and *Lie Que* (Lu 7) should be drained. If it is sunken, the condition is empty (*xu*). Therefore *Lie Que* (Lu 7) should be supplemented. It also clears phlegm from the chest, moistens a dry throat, and relieves cough. As the lung *luo* point, it has many effects which stem from the relationship between the paired internal/external channels. Therefore it can be used for intestinal troubles as well.

The lungs are related to the bladder. If the lung qi is full, it will hold fluids, causing slow or no urination. Therefore *Lie Que* (Lu 7) is used for prostate problems. But, if there is blood in the urine, drain *Lie Que* (Lu 7).

Because *Lie Que* (Lu 7) is a *luo* point, it is needled more on the yang side of the arm than are any of the other lung channel points. Avoid the blood vessel and direct the needle up the arm away from the hand, against the flow of the channel as draining is required in most cases.

He Gu (LI 4) has a close relationship with the triple heater channel which regulates the qi of the *san jiao* or 3 burners. Because of this, *He Gu* (LI 4) adjusts the whole body's activity or the *qi hua gong neng*, the qi transformation function and ability of the whole body, thus increasing the natural sources of healing power or righteous qi. As a large intestine channel point, it is especially able to increase movement below the navel.

The *yuan* source points of any of the 3 yang channels of the hand can be used to treat surface problems. All externally contracted cold diseases have yang channel treatments to let fever out. When the surface is tight or shut due to external cold congested in the skin and there is no perspiration, drain *He Gu* (LI 4) to expel the cold from the surface. The sensation should go up the arm until the pores open. Then perspiration will come out and the fever will go down. *He Gu* (LI 4) also has a special function of being able to clear external heat from the surface *and* it is used to treat cold, superficial emptiness conditions. This latter means that the surface is too loose and that the patient is perspiring too much already. In this case *He Gu* (LI 4) is supplemented by twirling the needle slightly. This closes the pores and sweat glands, clears heat, consolidates or astringes the skin, and stops perspiration.

He Gu (LI 4) and *Qu Chi* (LI 11) are the main points for treating all conditions of the head and face. The energy of *Qu Chi* (LI 11) goes on without stopping. The energy of *He Gu* (LI 4) rises and then scatters. When these two points are combined, they clear the heat and scatter wind. Therefore, they are used to eliminate upper burner heat. This action allows pure qi (*qing qi*) to float upward and thus combat colds and flu, upper respiratory tract infection, pneumonia and bronchitis. The head is the meeting place of all yang channels. The ears, eyes, mouth, nose, throat, all the sense orifices need pure or *qing qi* to function. Needling *He Gu* (LI 4) and *Qu Chi* (LI 11) ascends the pure or clear yang to the orifices, opening them and clearing the senses, scattering evil qi and opening circulation. Thus, the arisal of the clear to the head makes the whole body more full of energy since it is none other than the separation of clear and turbid by digestion or the spleen/stomach, the postnatal root of righteous qi.

From the preceding information it can be seen that among the points which comprise the formula which is the heart of this book *Zu San Li* (St 36) is the earth and *he* sea or uniting point of the stomach channel. *Qu Chi* (LI 11) is the earth and uniting point of the large intestine channel. *He Gu* (LI 4) and *Lie Que* (Lu 7) are the paired *yuan* source and *luo* connecting points of the large intestine and lungs. Only *San Yin Jiao* (Sp 6) has yet to be discussed.

E. Three Yin Crossing

San Yin Jiao (Sp 6) is not an antique point. It also has no five phase or transport designation. A distal point on the yin earth channel, it is in a special category all its own. Its name, *San Yin Jiao*, Three Yin Crossing, refers to the fact that the three yin channels of the leg cross at this point. While on the spleen channel, *San Yin Jiao* (Sp 6) connects with the kidney and liver qi as well. It controls yin blood in general and should usually be supplemented rather than drained.

One of *San Yin Jiao*'s main functions is to regulate the sexual and reproductive systems of both men and women. It has an especially powerful effect on the uterus since all three leg yin connect with the uterus. Stimulating it also restores the memory and helps the patient to feel younger and more alert because much of its power comes from its ability to strengthen kidney qi.

Because of its special function as the crossing point of the 3 leg yin, *San Yin Jiao*'s inclusion in the root formula described in this book means that all of the major yin organs of the body except the heart can be stimulated by this formula. However, when one treats the kidneys and the spleen, the heart is automatically regulated since the kidneys control the heart via the *ke* cycle and the spleen is the son of the heart according to the *sheng* cycle. (See Appendix B: The Heart and Kidney in Chinese Medicine)

F. Revival Points

Since ancient times certain points have been known to have a powerful effect on the body under conditions of extreme stress. The 9 which are considered the most potent are called "Revival Points". They are *San Yin Jiao* (Sp 6), *Lao Gong* (Per 8), *Zu San Li* (St 36), *Zhong Wan* (CV 12), *He Gu* (LI 4), *Huan Tiao* (GB 30), *Ya Men* (GV 15), *Yong Quan* (Ki 1), and *Tai Xi* (Ki 3).

The point combination which is the topic of this book includes three of these 9 points. There is little wonder then that this formula should have such a powerful effect in restoring strength to the body and to the spirit.

2

The Circulation of Qi & the Power of Distal Points

To understand Chinese medicine, the concept of balance is essential. The ideas of balance can be represented by a series of simple images and numerical relationships which, upon meditation and reflection, have a much deeper meaning.

The numbers 1, 3, 5, 7, and 9 represent yang energy. 0, 2, 4, 6, and 8 represent yin. Chinese medical theory defines health as the condition in which yin and yang energies in the body are balanced.

There are, however, many kinds of balance which can be symbolized by the arrangement of these numbers. One kind of balance, represented by the arrangement

$$-4, -3, -2, -1, =0= +1, +2, +3, +4$$

balances two numbers of like value but opposite sign to equal zero: -4 and +4 =0, etc. While -4 balances +4, this balance is static; the numbers cancel each other out. This is the kind of balance that occurs in death when yin and yang separate. There is no movement. So a dead man has arms and legs but cannot move; eyes, ears, brain, but cannot see, hear, or think.

The numerical configuration which represents life is based on 10:

$1 + 9 = 10$, $2 + 8$, $3 + 7$, and $4 + 6$ all equal 10. This configuration represents equilibrium but not perfect, static balance. There is movement. The changing combinations contribute to the sum of 10, which here represents life or health, the optimum interplay of all elements.

The ancients made a series of correspondences between these numerical configurations and the universe, both the macrocosm of earth and sky, weather and seasons, and the microcosm, the inner universe of each human being. Although this ancient Chinese science does not fit recent attempts to make traditional Chinese medicine look "scientific" according to the current Western definition, it still has great value. It provides a way for us to understand and utilize the energies of the human body through the points and channels of acupuncture and offers ways of envisioning interrelationships that we might otherwise miss.

In Chinese philosophy, the number 3 represents the west. Proceeding clockwise, the direction in which yang qi moves, $3 \times 3 = 9$, the north. Nine times $3 = 27$; 7 is the east. Seven times $3 = 21$; 1 represents the south. North plus south, and east plus west each equal 10. When 3, 7, 9, and 1 are added together they equal 20. Going in the opposite direction — counterclockwise or the direction of yin — begin from the northeast with 2. 2 times $2 = 4$; the northwest is 4. In the southwest, $4 \times 2 = 8$; $8 \times 2 = 16$, 6 is the southeast. Adding $2 + 4 + 6 + 8 = 20$. Only the number 5 remains unused. It is in the center of what is called the Magic Square.

4	9	2
3	5	7
8	1	6

In the universe, yang (the sky) equals 20. $20 \times 5 = 100$. Yin (the earth) also equals 20. $20 \times 5 = 100$. Both yin and yang are balanced, and all is well. In the Magic Square, if you add in any direction, horizontally, vertically, or diagonally, the total is 15. 15 is the number which represents human being who live between heave above and earth below.

As we mentioned in discussing the relationship of the yin and yang five phase points up the extremities, yin and yang within the human body must be balanced for health and growth. So too must the earth and sky be balanced for life to flourish. When earth and sky are in harmony, the climate is beneficial to human life. When the sky changes, the earth changes. When these changes are disharmonious, as in weather inappropriate to the season or excessive weather, humankind becomes sick. When the disharmonies are great, epidemics rage.

These patterns are borne out in clinical practice. Hot weather in late fall tends to bring on sore throats. When there are bitter cold, harsh winds too late in spring, the treatment rooms are filled with people with hip or neck and shoulder pain. Extreme, long periods of heat, cold, or rain leave even relatively strong patients vulnerable to problems to which they might not have succumbed under normal climatic conditions.

A. The Cause of Pain: Imbalances of Qi in the Body

The 6 qi or *liu qi* are the forces that effect the outer life of humankind which stem from the relationship of heaven and earth. These are cold, wind, wetness, dryness, heat, and summer heat. Also, within each human being is a small universe all its own. From this inner universe, *i.e.*, the relationships between the organs, and from family and interpersonal relationships come the 7 emotions: anger, fear, joy, grief, worry, sudden fright or shock, and melancholy.

When the inner universe is harmonious and the qi is strong and balanced, a person can ward off the disharmonies of the outer universe. When a person exhausts his or her righteous qi through excessive activity, irregular habits, overwork, or emotional exhaustion, this inner protection or righteous qi is depleted. Lowered resistance and frequent illness, emotional instability and pain result.

Imbalance may occur in the channels and connecting vessels *(jing luo)* or in the organs and bowels *(zang fu)*. As a rule, if the channel is in pain, treat one side. If the organ is involved treat both sides.

An example of the kind of channel pain that can result from invasion of external evil is the case of the overheated florist. Because he was too hot, he stuck his left arm in the freezer to cool himself off. The next day he could not move that arm. He had a "frozen shoulder" in more ways than one. The invasion of cold had blocked the flow of qi in the channels and connecting vessels of his arm leaving it immobile and in pain. This is based on the Chinese saying, "Where there is pain, there is no free flow."

Looking at the Magic Square as it might be superimposed on the body, 4 and 2 represent the locations of the shoulders, 2 being the side that had gotten chilled. Rather than treating the bad shoulder, I treated the good side, 4. We Chinese have a saying: "If the baby is sick, don't punish it."

When one area of the body lacks qi, there must be too much qi accumulated somewhere else. Because the body is symmetrical, the best place to look for the misplaced qi is on the opposite side. In the case of the florist mentioned above, I put a needle in his right shoulder, and had him work the left one until he could raise it again and the pain was less. This was accomplished by draining the full side to disperse the qi accumulated there. As the qi returns, the damaged side should begin to grow warmer. Having the patient move the affected side just to the point of pain, not beyond it, provides a signal to let the qi know where it is needed. After moving, the patient should stop and relax the area, allowing the qi to come in. Repeating this process every 10 minutes further opens the area, gradually restoring balance and the smooth flow of qi. It is possible too watch the patient become less tense and more mobile as the pain decreases. I feel that it is important, both for the patient and for me, to see and feel immediate results from the treatment.

Cupping the injured area for 10 minutes while the needles are in the opposite side adds to the effect of the treatment. Suction from the cups draws out stagnant blood and allows fresh, oxygenated blood to replace it. The combination of cups and needles promotes the return of both qi and blood to the area.

If treating the opposite side does not produce relief, I then look elsewhere for the full qi. One of the most powerful pathways by which the qi flows in the body is in a figure eight:

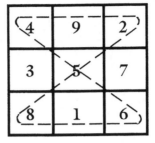

Therefore, another possibility, using the Magic Square, would be to treat 8, or the position on opposite side and below, since the problem is above, in this case, the opposite leg. I would use *Yang Ling Quan* (GB 34). In addition to being in the right location diagonal to the problem, *Yang Ling Quan* (GB 34) is a special point for the *jin* or tendons and ligaments.

Following the figure 8 superimposed on the Magic Square, if one goes diagonally from any problem, it is easy to find a point which will treat that problem successfully.

B. Using the Circulation of Qi for the Treatment of Both Local Conditions & Systemic Imbalances

The effect of treatment at a distance from the problem can be represented in another way. A physical representation of the action of this principle is the configuration of four balls hung by string from a frame. It looks like this:

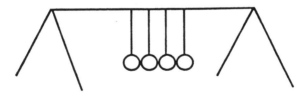

When the ball on one end is swung into the adjacent one, it imparts its impact without moving the second and then the third balls very far. The force can be seen only when it reaches the last ball, which when knocked by the third ball swings as widely as did the first one. Needling the feet to treat the hands or head or needling the hands or head to treat the feet is a clinical application of the principle of the circulation of qi. Based on this idea, when there is a headache, one can often treat the feet at *Shen Mai* (Bl 62) and *Jin Men* (Bl 63) or *Yong Quan* (Ki 1). Or, if the soles of the feet hurt, one may treat *Bai Hui* (GV 20).[4] When the back of the neck is heavy and the patient has high blood pressure, treat the feet, *i.e.*, *Yong Quan* (Ki 1), applying yin to control yang. Painful soles are due to a lack of yin energy. Treat yang to protect yin.

Other examples of treating distant from the point of pain or disease include treating *Xing Jian* (Liv 2) for jaw pain. For eye problems one can use 4 special points called "Flower Bone 1" along the underside of the foot, between the great and second toe directly below the liver channel. These points are very useful. (See Appendix D for illustrations of extra points.) These treatments follow the principles of the circulation of qi that if the qi in the head is over-active, drain on the feet. If there is too little qi, supplement the distal points. If pain is one-sided, treat the opposite side. If as in red, itchy, tearing eyes, both sides are involved, use Flower Bone 1 on both feet. Jaw pain is usually a channel problem. Eye problems generally indicate imbalance of the liver organ.

C. Using the Circulation of Qi for Treating Systemic Imbalances

When the patient comes with a problem in which the functioning of the whole body is involved as opposed to simply localized impairment, it may necessary to draw on more channels and to tap both yin and yang qi. Because the spleen and stomach are the root of production of righteous qi which nourishes all the organs and the lungs and large intestine command the defensive or *wei qi* at the surface of the body, the use of points on these 4 channels greatly strengthens the patient's resistance to outside influences

---

[4]   If the feet are painful, use *Jian Yu* (LI 15).

and assists the functioning of the internal organs. In this case, treatment is given bilaterally to points above and below.

3

Selecting Channels for Treatment & Using the 24 Hour Chinese Clock

Knowing the time that a symptom occurs sometimes helps in determining its source or choosing the channel to treat. In other cases, time is less a factor than the symptom itself. The following 2 cases illustrate methods for choosing the channel to treat based on the circulation of qi and the Chinese biorhythmic clock.

Case 1

A heavy woman in her 50's had for two years had a severe case of flatulence. She passed gas only after 11 AM and all afternoon until 6 PM. I could not picture how the time of occurrence related to her trouble. Often intestine trouble happens at large intestine time — 7-9 AM. This woman's flatulence, however, occurred at heart, small intestine, bladder and kidney time, according to the Chinese clock (see diagram).

I told her to buy doves' eggs and eat 2 at a time each day for 3 days, but she could not find them. Therefore she came for treatment even though she was very afraid of needles. I used *Nei Ting* (St 44) and *Xian Gu* (St 43) on the left foot. (Left for women, right for men in the afternoon. In the morning, reverse sides treating women on the right, etc.) After one treatment, her husband came and told me that her trouble had stopped, but she did not want to come back for fear of the needles. I got her to return for one more treatment. That was 1½ years ago and she has had no further trouble since then. This treatment works according to the pattern by which qi flows through the body:

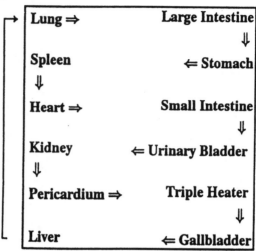

Using this pattern of flow through the 12 regular channels, it is possible to treat in either direction. One can use large intestine points for stomach problems or stomach points for large intestine problems. This is an example of yang to treat yang. It is also possible to use yin to treat yang, for instance using lung for large intestine problems, or yang to treat yin, stomach points for spleen problems.

I liken this to the way people are when they are upset. Sometimes you need to talk to your husband or wife or a close friend or relative of the opposite sex. Sometimes, though, a man must get the advice of another man, or a woman the support of another woman. Choosing channels follows the same patterns.

In this treatment, once I had chosen the channel, *i.e.*, the stomach to treat the large intestine or yang to treat yang, I selected the points on the channel according to five phase theory. *Xian Gu* (St 43) is the wood point on the stomach channel. Gas is a kind of wind, wind being related to liver wood. In this case, wood is insulting metal or the liver rebelling against the large intestines. *Nei Ting* (St 44) is the water point and water is the mother of wood. Treating *Nei Ting* (St 44) harmonizes and nourishes wood through its effect on water. These points are also helpful for diarrhea with abdominal pain and for people whose bowels move soon after every meal.

Combining two points on the same channel increases the efficacy of the treatment. Also, some patients feel that only one needle could not possibly be enough even if that point is the perfect bull's eye point; so using two reassures them.

When you add times to the previously-mentioned energy flow chart, you have the Chinese biorhythmic clock. It is used when symptoms reoccur at a specific time as Case 2 illustrates. When the Chinese clock is added to the circulation of qi through the 12 regular channels it looks like this:

Lung (3-5 AM)⇒	Large Intestine (5-7 AM) ⇓
Spleen (9-11 AM) ⇓	⇐ Stomach (7-9 AM)
Heart (11AM-1PM) ⇒	Small Intestine (1-3 PM) ⇓
Kidney (5-7 PM) ⇓	⇐ Urinary Bladder (3-5 PM)
Pericardium (7-9 PM) ⇒	Triple Heater (9-11 PM) ⇓
Liver (1-3 AM)	⇐ Gallbladder (11 PM- 1AM)

These are the times when each channel has the most qi within a normal 24 hour day. Problems in the channels often manifest themselves at these times.

Case 2

A man had been having right-sided headaches for 3 years. They always began at 12:23 AM during gall bladder channel time. He had been treated in a Chinese clinic for 3 months. By needling points on his head, the acupuncturist could alleviate the pain but for only a few hours. It always returned. Sometimes the frontal part of the headache would go away but occipital pain would remain or the pain would shift from front to back after treatment.

This is one of the drawbacks of using only points located near the problem. In solely local treatment for headache, there is nothing to anchor the qi and draw it downward out of the head. Some residual pain always remains as does the tendency for the headache to return full force. Treatment of points in the lower extremities provides this downward motion, stabilizing the energy much more effectively.

When I treated this patient, I gave him the special point on inch below *Yang Ling Quan* (GB 34), *Da Nang Xue* (M-LE-23), and a second point 2 inches below that on the left leg. These points I call Beside Three Miles because the upper point is located just lateral to *Zu San Li* (St 36).

In my office in the United States, I usually leave these needles in for 45 minutes. In China, the treatments only last 3 minutes because there are so many people waiting and only a few beds available. I left the needle in for 10 minutes, at the end of which time the pain was gone. I told the man to return every day for the next 4 days. When he came back the day after the first treatment, the headache had not returned. That was the only treatment I gave him and for the next 4 days that I was visiting that city, his pain did not return.

I chose these points because the pain happened at gall bladder channel time. For a right-sided headache, I needle the left leg according to the figure 8 pattern of qi flow on the Magic Square. The location of this headache was between the bladder, gall bladder and stomach channels and not clearly on any one channel. When a problem crosses 2 or more channels, I use special points rather than standard channel points. The principle of needling 2 points on the same channel for amplification of stimulation has already been discussed.

4

Earth as Center

The Magic Square which we used to represent the flow of qi from one end of the body to the other can also be used as a way to see the possibilities of regulating the body's qi from the center.

While the five phases are generally represented like this:

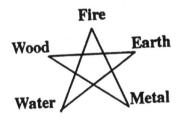

In order to portray their relationships in the cycles of generation and control, they can also be represented thus:

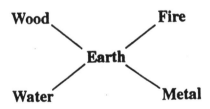

So it is in the Magic Square. The earth phase, represented by the number 5, is in the center of the square. Through it, all other numbers, representing all other organs, can be reached and regulated. The power of the earth phase to regulate the rest of the phases and qi will be made clear in the case histories and explanations of the clinical applications of *Zu San Li* (St 36), *San Yin Jiao* (Sp

6), *He Gu* (LI 4), *Qu Chi* (LI 11), and *Lie Que* (Lu 7) which follow in Section 2.

The importance of the functioning of earth or the spleen and stomach, middle burner of *zhong jiao* cannot be over-emphasized. It is responsible for the production of all qi which comes to the body after birth.[5]

If the nutritional intake is inadequate or improper, the spleen and stomach will not have the fuel they need to power and restore the body. The original qi, which is the body's reserve, is drawn on until it too is used up, thus leaving the patient weak and exhausted, unable to handle stress or fight off disease. Emotional instability or susceptibility to infection, and particularly respiratory infection, follow. Because earth generates metal, the spleen is the mother of the lungs. Therefore, weakness in earth leads to problems in metal.

If a patient becomes faint when needled, the first question to ask if whether they have eaten. Acupuncture uses the patient's own qi for healing. If the stomach is empty, the qi the needles tap will be their own original qi. If that patient is very weak, this will leave them weak and faint. Needling can drain the patient's qi even when supplementation technique is used. If one has eaten recently, one will have qi available from the food, and it is this the needles can tap. However, if the patient has just eaten a heavy meal, their energy will be so involved in the process of digestion that it will be unavailable then as well. Ideally the patient should eat a moderate meal some 60 minutes before receiving acupuncture.

It is also important for the patient to eat at a reasonable time after receiving a treatment. Continuing activity with no nourishment after strong acupuncture stimulation can result in extreme fatigue.

---

[5] At birth the individual receives original or *yuan* qi from their parents. This original qi is stored in the kidneys and is regulated by using *San Yin Jiao* (Sp 6).

5

The Lungs' Anti-Gravitational Function in Chinese Physiology

As the highest located organ in the torso, the lungs are responsible for raising and holding up the qi, fluids, and the solid aspects of the body. Their qi, when functioning properly, works much like a dip tube. A simple experiment with a straw will demonstrate this principle. Put one end of the straw into a glass of liquid. Then hold one finger over the top of the straw so that it is completely covered. When the straw is removed from the glass, whatever liquid was in the straw will remain there, held by atmospheric pressure pushing up on the bottom of the straw. If the finger is removed from the top, the atmospheric pressure is equal on the top and bottom of the straw and the force of gravity is then able to draw the liquid down.

The lungs have a similar anti-gravitational action in the body. When lung qi is too low, the nose runs. Older women often find themselves releasing urine when they laugh or sneeze. And in situations of great fear, people lose control of urination and bowel movement. Excessive tearing, drooling, or perspiration may also occur depending on which other organs are also effected—tearing relates to liver, drooling to spleen, perspiration to heart, urinary incontinence to kidney. When lung qi is full or (shi), there is difficult or no urination. The qi is too strong to allow appropriate flow. Poor circulation, on the other hand, as evidenced by purple or bluish color of the extremities and particularly the toes, in indicative of lung weakness. The lung qi is unable to bring the blood back to the heart.

According to five phase theory, metal produces water. Therefore, the lungs are the mother of the kidneys. Thus, for kidney emptiness, supplement the lungs. Because fire melts metal, thinking too much, one of the causes of heart fire, damages the lungs which then cannot nourish the kidneys. Dehydration of all tissues results if the condition continues over time.

One more theory is necessary to our understanding of the power of the points selected for the formula under discussion.

6

Stomach & Large Intestine Channels Have More Qi & More Blood

According to traditional Chinese theory, each of the channels has its own resources of qi and blood. To a great degree, the strengths of action and spheres of influence of the points have to do with the amount of qi and/or blood available in their respective channels. Points on those channels which have both more qi and more blood can safely be supplemented or drained as much as necessary without throwing other organs out of balance or depleting the whole system. As can be seen from the chart on the following page, the stomach and large intestine channels, collectively referred to as the *yang ming*, are the only 2 of the 12 regular channels which have both more qi and more blood. In this chart "+" means more, "—" means less.

Channel	Qi	Blood
Lung	+	—
Large Intestine	+	+
Stomach	+	+
Spleen	+	—
Heart	+	—

Small Intestine	—	+
Bladder	—	+
Kidney	+	—
Pericardium	—	+
Triple Heater	+	—
Gall Bladder	+	—
Liver	—	+

Section 2

The Clinical Applications of *Zu San Li* (St 36), *San Yin Jiao* (Sp 6), *He Gu* (LI 4), *Qu Chi* (LI 11), & *Lie Que* (Lu 7):

One Combination of Points Can Treat Many Diseases

1

Intention & Healing the Patient, Not Just the Disease

I have explained why I have chosen the points in this formula in terms of their individual characteristics. In combination, these points are balanced in terms of yin and yang and in their locations on both upper and lower extremities and are used bilaterally. These factors, in addition to the combined effect of their individual functions, give them the power to regulate the overall functioning of the body.

The cases in this section show how this formula can be used for systemic problems and Western diseases such as depression, hypertension, and allergies. To treat systemic problems, which are often chronic, the acupuncturist must have correct technique, a proper understanding of the on-going sources of disease, and a clearly focused intention for the patient to get well which must be communicated, one way or another, to the patient.

Specifics regarding technique are included in this chapter, as well as my understanding of the causes of the imbalances which result in systemic disease. While acupuncture can rebalance the body's qi, if there are major disharmonies in the patient's emotional habits or lifestyle which continue to disrupt his or her qi, treatment results may not be as thorough, long-lasting, or powerful as we would like them to be.

In Chinese medicine, we seek to treat the problem at its root, addressing not just the symptoms but their underlying causes. When a patient comes with pain due to blockage of a channel, one or only a few treatment may solve the problem completely and it may not recur for years if ever. Organ imbalances are deeper. They typically are the result of long years of mismanaging one's qi, and the treatment too must go deeper and take longer.

Therefore, we must address not only the causes of disease but also the ways to health. Knowing how to maintain qi in going from sickness to greater health and knowing how to maintain a healthy, balanced life in the face of the world and all its pressures is no small accomplishment. People who live long, active lives have a system. No matter how busy, how sad or joyous or upset, they know their limits. The do not go beyond what their bodies can take.

It is often possible to get rid of pain or internal imbalance for a time by considering the patient only, by working with the qi which they have available at the moment of treatment. But preventing further trouble and restoring health is another matter entirely. To prevent disease and re-establish vitality, both the acupuncturist and the patient must use the whole universe wisely.

There are patterns by which the people living in different cultures abuse their energies, and in each country, patients have different expectations of what an acupuncturist has to offer. Patients in the United States, especially younger ones, are much more likely than Chinese people to come in saying, "I come here and pay you to treat me. Make me well but don't expect me to change the way I live. Just fix me." As though their bodies were machines for which I could provide new parts.

We have an old saying in China: "When you are under 30, you can cheat disease. When you are over 30, disease cheats you." One important aspect of practicing Chinese medicine is helping people to see how they are cheating themselves out of health. Holding the firm and clear intention that the patient can overcome the illness is a crucial part of treatment. That matter of intention is discussed in a later section.

2

Depression &
Running on Empty

Depression is one of the most serious unseen diseases in America. Most doctors do not know how to treat it, but from my many years of experience with American patients, I have found a way that works well.

Depression attacks slowly, unnoticed. It begins with small unhappinesses in the family or at work, problems so small one can't express them even to oneself. These unhappinesses accumulate over the years. After 5—10 years, the person has grown weaker and weaker. Then, any strong emotional upset or setback in life may bring on a severe attack of depression.

In the United States, family problems are due to the fact that both husband and wife are engaged in too many individual activities. Each has his or her own car. They may have their own beds or even their own rooms and separate finances. After they quarrel, they can drive off in their cars or shut themselves up in their rooms. Becoming increasingly disharmonious and distant, they may separate completely. In the body, when yin and yang separate, death results. In marriage, when yin and yang or husband and wife separate, they relationship "breaks up", and the family is split. But divorce is not an end to the emotional problems that can be generated when man and woman pull apart instead of together. They must still divide their property and their children, and so the process continues.

In China there is one bedroom and one blanket. When the couple quarrels, there is nowhere else to go. They must eventually come together and touch each other, and this helps to dissolve the tension. Traditionally, when roles were set, with the husband going to work and the wife managing the home, the pressures of daily activity were less on both. In a traditional household, the yin tasks and the yang tasks are completed. One person does not have to do or be everything. The husband earns the money; the wife does not have to do so. The wife makes a clean, warm home where the husband can rest after work. She makes sure there is always strengthening food prepared so that her husband and children will be sustained. Man and woman need each other, and this brings the family together.

On my visits to China, people often say to me that they wish they could live in the United States where people have so much. They cannot know what I see here. Everyone is exhausted, especially the women, who must not only manage the home and raise the children but must earn a living as well. Not only this, but in addition, many people here feel they need to get more training to get a better job if they are to get ahead or just keep up, so when they return tired from work, they stay up late to study. Exhausted, the stresses of their lives may seem overwhelming and depression sets in.

Depression in China is much more due to politics. Parents worry about their teenagers having no schools in which to study or that they will be sent to the countryside to be farmers. Even if a person works for 20 — 30 years, their salary will not increase. There is no housing, no promotions. A salary cut may lead to suicide. Anger is greater in China. There is more obvious unfairness. There is much high cholesterol, heart disease and stroke, not from rich food, which is limited, but because of frustration and depression.

In the U.S., the problem is not one of limitation but of the lack of limits. People work hard and then play hard. They can go anywhere, do anything, have anything that their credit allows. This is different than only doing what their true financial situation allows. Many people are in debt, living beyond their means. They are also in debt physically and emotionally, living beyond their energetic means. Because they play as hard as they work, and travel, sometimes frantically on their vacations, they never truly rest. Exhausted, they do not have the reserves to deal with the stresses of life. Forever engaged in yang activities, there is neither the commitment nor knowledge of how to nourish the yin which is necessary to the rebuilding of true or *zhen* yang.

Many of the people I see lack true nourishment. Instead of well-cooked, carefully planned meals appropriate to the season which are eaten slowly and in a relaxed manner, Americans often substitute fast foods eaten on the run. Such foods have had all their vitality removed. Those who are "health-conscious" supplement their diets with vitamins and minerals, but from the standpoint of Chinese medicine, such supplements supply instant energy of a false yang nature. Rather than nourishing true qi, it feeds what we call empty fire and pushes them further beyond their actual limits.

Most people know that stimulants such as amphetamines and cocaine are harmful. But they do not realize that they are using their vitamins to perpetuate the same cycle of overextension. Neither they nor those who use coffee, chocolate, sugar, and cigarettes wish to recognize that they too are using powerful drugs to increase their energy. Overstimulated, they are unable to rest when rest is appropriate. They may use alcohol, marijuana, and tranquilizers to sedate the anxiety, tenseness, and irritability that are symptoms of both running on empty and taking stimulants. Rather than helping the problem, these substances further contribute to empty fire.

Many Americans are without a center in the sense that they have no centering, grounding focus for their choices and actions emotionally and in the sense that they have, through neglect and abuse, damaged the physical center of their life's energy—earth or the spleen/stomach whose vital importance in Chinese medicine has already been mentioned.

The patient either becomes hyper in his activities, working non-stop, working and then going out with friends, or exercising frantically. Or they become depressed, or both. Digestion and appetite are affected, and the person generally has trouble sleeping. Long term insomnia depletes yin and increases internal heat. Tossing and turning, disturbing dreams, and further loss of sleep result, producing more empty heat in a vicious circle. This heat enters the lungs and large intestine. Thus the stools harden, peristalsis is inhibited, and constipation results.

As the person becomes more depressed and exhausted, their lung qi becomes weaker. The lungs' function, as has been mentioned above, is to work against gravity. The characteristic of its qi is to pull upward, holding the body and its fluids against the downward pull of the earth's gravitation. When the lung qi is strong, the person can think, walk, hold and see things, can stand and act. If lung qi is lowered due to unnoticed depression creeping in, the person slowly begins to feel lazy or lethargic. They may like to lie down more and think less, get less exercise, and experience difficulty making plans and decisions.

In Western physiological terms, a decrease in respiration and over-all metabolism brings less and less oxygen to the brain. As the brain lacks the oxygen it requires to function, changes take place in the vital endocrine glands housed within it. These glands, which Chinese medical theory long recognized functionally as "internal secretion" while not identifying their anatomical structures, regulate the functioning of the entire organism.

Case 1: Depression & Heart Qi

A well dressed woman came to her physician, who is a friend of mine. I was visiting at the time and sat in on her appointment. She complained of a general feeling that she was not well. A social worker by profession, she had to decide who was to receive benefits and who should not. Some families she could help, some she had to cut off. Those who received aid praised her, those whom she found ineligible cursed her. She held up under this pressure with dignity and continued to do her best. When I felt her pulses, they lacked yang qi and I said to her, "You are depressed." At this she began to cry, unable to hold back her tears. I had touched the inner, hidden disease. According to five phase theory, this is considered to be a case of heart heat, evil heat building from the stresses at her job, invading or over-controlling lung metal. Thus weakened, the lungs could not hold back her tears. (See Appendix B on the role of the heart in Chinese medicine.)

This woman also suffered burning urination. When the heat in the heart goes to its paired organ, the small intestine, burning urination results. This is explained by the fact that qi circulates from the small intestine to the bladder. Heat in the small intestine will manifest in bladder symptoms such as frequent, painful, urgent, burning urination.

The patient also had alternating constipation and diarrhea and had been diagnosed as having diverticulitis. While alternating constipation and diarrhea also relate to the small intestine, the weakening and stretching of the smooth muscle walls of the large intestine show that the heart, burning with too much evil heat, was unable to nourish the spleen. Fire generates earth but too much fire fails to produce earth. The spleen rules the flesh and muscles. When it is strong, the flesh and muscles or *ji rou* of the body have good tone and are able to support themselves and other tissues.

I therefore supplemented *Zu San Li* (St 36), drained *He Gu* (LI 4) and *Lie Que* (Lu 7), but as I was visiting and she was not my patient, I could only give her one treatment.

Case 2: Depression & Lung Qi

In 1974 I was very busy. Early one morning, about 6:30 AM, 4 large business men brought another man into my office. They dragged him in and made him lie down. One of the 4 whispered to me that their friend had tried to commit suicide 4 times. He had lost money in business and had trouble with women. His pulse was very weak, lacking yang qi. He had no desire to go on or to do anything to help himself.

To the Chinese understanding, each organ houses an aspect of spirit. Considered to be different types of souls, these aspects have different names and properties. The souls housed in the liver and spleen go upward to heaven after death. The soul housed in the lungs is not spirit, but knowledge and activity which the person has acquired during his lifetime: knowledge of how to make a living, how to make one's way in the world against all the forces which would sweep on aside. As the lung qi works physically in the body against the force of gravity to hold up tears, etc., so too lung qi on an emotional or soul level holds up the spirit against the gravity of our struggle to survive in the world. When the lung qi is low, that knowledge of how to live becomes weaker and may be lost. When this soul goes, the person's will to live is gone.

Healthy fish swim upstream against the current. Only hurt or dead fish wash ashore. The gravity of the earth tries to pull us down as well as nourishing us. For this reason, it is not enough to merely supplement earth in a case of such severe depression. The lung qi must be increased as well. So for this patient I also gave *Zu San Li* (St 36), *He Gu* (LI 4), and *Lie Que* (Lu 7).

41

Zu San Li (St 36) is the *he* sea point. It increases digestion, helps the body to absorb food, increases the production of gastric acids, and stimulates hunger. I needle it first because it tranquilizes the patient and protects them against fainting reaction to the needles. It increases the flow of energy and oxygen to the head since the stomach channel begins on the head. When needling the stomach channel on the feet, all the qi is sent upward. After stimulating *Zu San Li* (St 36), you can see the face become infused with redness, glowing and warm.

Technique is very important. I put in both needles and then *de qi* or obtain the qi. Then, with my right hand on the needle in the left leg and my left hand on the needle in the right leg, with the needles inserted shallowly, I move both thumbs forward 240 degrees and backwards 120 degrees or ⅔ of a full turn around forward and ⅓ turn back. This is done 3 times and then the needle is thrust a little deeper, turned as above 3 times, again thrust deeper and turned 3 times, for a total of 9 turns. It is important that both needles be turned at the same time.

Depth at the various stages of insertion is determined by dividing the final needle depth by 3. For example, the range of depth of insertion for *Zu San Li* (St 36) is 1–2 inches according to the Shang Hai College of TCM acupuncture text. At times I needle it deeper, selecting the depth according to the musculature of the patient. This man was large. Therefore I went in first ¾ inch, then 1½ inches, and then 2¼ inches.

Repeat the turnings 9 times until the propagation of qi reaches the toes. If the qi moves only to the ankle, it will stick there and the patient will experience difficulty walking and moving that ankle after the treatment. The qi must go to the toes. After the qi has reached the end of the channel, pull the needle up above the channel and above the muscle but not out of the skin and leave it shallow, pointing in the direction the channel flows. In the case of the stomach channel, point it towards the foot. This is the technique for supplementation.

The next needle I used on this distraught man was *He Gu* (LI 4) to strengthen his lung qi. Because the lungs and large intestine are paired organs according to the husband-wife law of acupuncture, it is possible to use the *biao* or external organ of a pair to treat the *li* or internal organ. To strengthen the lungs, *He Gu* (LI 4) is drained.

The reason for using drainage or *xie fa* is this: The lungs are rarely empty or deficient in the true sense but are usually filled with evil qi which has developed there in the absence of righteous qi. This evil qi stagnates and transforms into heat.[6]

Lung qi works differently from the qi of other organs. It is innervated by the sympathetic rather than the parasympathetic nervous system. Usually we think of supplementing for weak qi, but, in the lungs, we must drain evil heat. With the evil heat removed, the true energy of the lungs automatically increases. In fact, supplementing the lungs reduces their true qi. Therefore, it is dangerous to supplement *He Gu* (LI 4) on pregnant women unless it is time to help her deliver. At this time *He Gu* (LI 4) is supplemented to drain the qi of the lungs so that the lungs will release the fetus to the downward force of gravity.

In the case of the patient who had tried to commit suicide, I also used *Lie Que* (Lu 7) to increase the effect of *He Gu* (LI 4) and to strengthen the large intestine. The man had come in quietly, refusing to talk, and he left after the half–hour treatment without saying a word. The next day, 2 men brought him, but still he said nothing. The third day, only one man came with him and he said "Hello". On the fourth day, he came alone and spoke to the other patients. On the fifth day, (I treated him 5 days in a row) he stayed after the treatment and talked to people in the office. He did not return the next week. I believe he was recovered.

In Chinese theory, if the lungs are weak, supplement earth, the mother, in order to strengthen metal, the son. *Zu San Li* (St 36) is the major distal supplementation point for earth.

---

[6]

It is mentioned in the *Nei Jing* that a condition of heat and dryness in the lungs will soften the legs, as in multiple sclerosis, so that the patient cannot walk.

Clinically, it is more powerful in its effect that *Jie Xi* (St 41) which is the fire or mother point on the stomach channel. *Jie Xi* (St 41) is the point that would be chosen according to a strict application of the mother-son law of five phase theory. There are obviously many ways to interpret and employ this theory. To my way of thinking, a flexible application is best or one which takes advantage of other experience, such as the fact that *Zu San Li* (St 36) is one of the most powerful supplementation points of the entire body.

Hand or Needle Technique

Hand technique for supplementation of all channels whose qi goes from the top down, *i.e.*, the stomach, bladder, gallbladder channels on the leg and the heart, lungs, and pericardium channels on the arm, is thumbs forward when both needles are turned simultaneously, the practitioner's right hand on the needle in the patient's left side, etc. For channels which run from the toes or finger to the chest or head, *i.e.* the liver, spleen, kidneys, large intestine, triple heater, small intestine, use the opposite technique for supplementation or thumbs backward.

For drainage, simply reverse this hand technique or *shou fa*. Therefore, to drain *He Gu* (LI 4), with the right hand on the needle in the left side of the patient's body and the left hand on the needle in the right side, move the thumbs forward. In addition, when draining, place the needle deeper upon insertion, move the thumb forward ⅓ turn and back ⅔ turn 3 times, then pull the needle up and repeat the 3 turns for a total of 6 turns. Then push the needle deep until one obtains the qi and leave it at this depth pointing against the flow of the channel. In the case of *He Gu* (LI 4), it should be directed slightly back toward the fingertips. *Lie Que* (Lu 7) is turned in the opposite direction from *Zu San Li* (St 36) because *Zu San Li* (St 36) is being supplemented and *Lie Que* (Lu 7) is being drained. The needle is pointed up the arm, against the flow of the channel.

The efficacy of acupuncture depends on *de qi* or obtaining the qi. In cases of depression, it is difficult to obtain this sensation because the patient's qi is depressed and empty. If you do not *de qi* on the first attempt, leave the needles in, wait, rest, and then repeat the stimulation, possibly needling deeper, and send your own qi in through the needles to the patient.

When one cannot *de qi*, the patient feels no qi travelling from the needles, only soreness. It is important for the patient to understand the significance of the sensation you are seeking so that they can bear with the discomfort of the stimulation. You must watch the patient's reactions closely to make sure they have experienced *de qi*. Often, when you *de qi*, the patient will jump and then relax. During the stimulation which leads to *de qi*, it is much better if the patient can relax into the sensation rather than tightening up his or her muscles to try to ward off pain. Tenseness increases the pain and blocks the flow of qi.

As soon as the needle stimulation obtains the qi, the patient usually sighs deeply, drawing more air into their body. This indicates that some of the blockage has been released. It is like opening a vacuum jar. Pure air rushes in. The patient may then fall asleep. This is a good sign and is an indication that they may recover quickly.

Case 3: Depression & Spleen Qi

A woman had 2 sons who were both sent to Viet Nam during the war. For 2 years she worried night and day. She could not eat or sleep but prayed constantly. Gradually, all her muscles became loose and soft like jello. She could not move her arms and legs. She could not walk. Even when her 2 sons returned safely from the war, the joy she felt could not heal her. She was over 60 at the time, and the damage was very severe. While we could treat her, recovery could not be rapid or complete.

This is an extreme example of the way in which depression and worry affect the spleen. Because the spleen rules the flesh and muscles, often we see severely depressed patients who cannot even lift their arms to comb their hair and mildly depressed patients who complain that they feel heavy and sluggish and "just can't seem to get moving". After treatment with the points under discussion, she was able to regain much of her lost strength.

Case 4: Depression & Liver Qi

This condition often occurs in older women whose children are grown and have left home. Though on good terms with her husband, one woman I treated had found herself crying for hours and muttering for no apparent reason. Even she could not explain why.

Here, because the spleen had been weakened, the liver overcontrolled it and also insulted the lungs which could then no longer hold back the tears. Using the point combination *Zu San Li* (St 36), *He Gu* (LI 4), and *Lie Que* (Lu 7) increases lung qi in order to control liver wood. There may also be hidden anger stimulating the liver. The benefit of this treatment can be increased if the acupuncturist can somehow help the patient to recognize and deal with such unknown or unacknowledged feelings.

Because the woman in this instance was in her 60's, one month's treatment was necessary to strengthen and bring her organs back into balance. I also added *San Yin Jiao* (Sp 6) to help the reproductive organs, to regulate hormones, to retard aging since kidney qi rules internal secretion and regulates the aging process, and to calm the liver. *Qu Chi* (LI 11), another *he* sea point, was also included as it helps digestion and absorption when it is combined with *San Yin Jiao* (Sp 6) and *Zu San Li* (St 36).

I have always held that the fewer needles, the better the treatment — when they are the right needles. And so, in the evolution of this point formula, I initially began with *Zu San Li* (St 36), *He Gu* (LI 4) and *Lie Que* (Lu 7) only, adding *San Yin Jiao* (Sp 6) and *Qu Chi* (LI 11) when extra strengthening seemed necessary. As time went on, however, I realized that almost all patients in need of the first 3 points also needed the other 2 points. Therefore this formula came to include all 5 points.

Depression & Kidney Qi

As has been mentioned, kidney qi regulates the aging process. When a young person overworks and does not rest, cannot sleep well, becomes forgetful, and their hair grays prematurely or falls out, this is a sign of depression involving the kidneys. Using the 5 point formula is especially important in this case.

3

Multiple Sclerosis

Multiple sclerosis is often related to long term or habitual irregular eating, tension, and emotions which affect the appetite. Excessive emotional upset harms the liver and causes it to overcontrol the spleen. Nourishment which should be supplied by the spleen is not available, and the kidneys' stored resources are depleted. In Chinese physiology, the kidneys control the brain and spinal cord while the liver is associated with the nerves.

When poor nutrition and emotional tension have depleted the righteous qi which maintains all the tissues of the body, any intense disappointment, emotional, or physical trauma can trigger a more severe and rapid deterioration. This process may be likened to the way in which a worm eats away at a leaf. With its structure weakened, the leaf more easily breaks off in a storm than it would if it had been intact. Because the person's qi has been lowered and its circulation impaired, not enough oxygen reaches the brain, the internal secretions and the cerebro-spinal fluid change, and the myelin sheaths of the nerves degenerate.

In addition to using *Zu San Li* (St 36), *San Yin Jiao* (Sp 6), *He Gu* (LI 4), *Qu Chi* (LI 11), and *Lie Que* (Lu 7), the *Hua To Jia Ji* points must be used to help increase the circulation of the cerebrospinal fluid. Patients receiving strong stimulation of these points along the spine can feel qi moving down the spine and out to the extremities. The points are stimulated with a 7 star hammer. Hammer directly on the spine and on the inner bladder line as well or needle bilaterally, one after the other, down the spine. After this treatment, patients find themselves more awake and alert, relaxed and with more strength in their arms and legs. Treatment should be given daily for 1–3 weeks, then 3 times weekly, then twice, then once a week, tapering down gradually as the patient's response improves. In the beginning, changes in strength and motility last only 1 day. Then they will last for 2, then a week, a month, until recovery. But it takes many treatments and a strong commitment to changing lifestyle, diet, and emotional habits as well.

Case 5: Numbness, Possible Multiple Sclerosis

A woman aged 40 came to the clinic because her fingers, particularly the little ones, had been numb for 2 months. Western medical diagnosis had indicated the possibility of multiple sclerosis in its early stages. According to Western medicine, the cause of MS is uncertain. It is difficult to diagnose until its later stages, and no specific therapy is known.

For the previous 2 years, the patient had experienced a period of intense depression, anger, and sadness following the ending of a relationship. A smoker, her tongue was covered with thick, yellow fur. Her knees were mottled red and her toes were red, signs of poor circulation due partly to her smoking and partly to the way her qi was locked up in unresolved feelings. She also had hypoglycemia.

Because numbness can be aggravated by cold, she was advised to stop eating salads and other raw food and to avoid cold or iced drinks. However, excessive emotions, especially those associated with a broken heart, sadness, anger, depression, worry, constant replay of mental dialogues — "he said . . ., I said . . ." — were the deeper root of her problem. These mental dialogues are destructive, never-ending loops that can bind up a person's qi with a chain as strong as iron and consume it with nothing to show but suffering. When this internal dialogue takes over, the patient cannot concentrate, cannot sleep, may eat a lot and gain no weight or may eat little and add pounds, all indications of internal secretion imbalance. Eventually, muscle control is lost and coordination is impaired.

As mentioned previously, acupuncture can restore some amount of control once it has been lost but requires many sessions over a long period of time. If the syndrome is recognized and dealt with early, the worst effects can be averted and the body's fuller utilization of its qi can be restored in a course of treatment 2 times a week for several weeks.

Upon first application of *Zu San Li* (St 36), this patient released a great sigh. Often such unhappy patients, particularly women, will be heard to sigh frequently, long and loudly. This is an attempt to release the blocked qi which has built up, but as the blockages are deeply rooted, sighing alone cannot release them. I added *He Gu* (LI 4), *Lie Que* (Lu 7) and indirectly moxaed *Shan Zhong* (CV 17). Moxa at this point was a very important part of the treatment in this case. It opens blocked qi and adds qi and warmth to the depressed system. *Shan Zhong* (CV 17) is the *hui* reunion point of the qi and the front *mu* point of the pericardium channel — the *jue yin* channel paired with the liver. It opens qi congestion in the chest. The patient will sigh deeply during the treatment, but, with the passages opened by the needles, she will be able to release more deeply and completely.

Though treatment can help to break the blockages of the energy, the patient herself must decide to step out of the circle of thoughts and memories, hurt, anger, guilt, and resentment. Acupuncture treatment can increase the qi available to make these changes in dealing with life's problems and thus change the vicious downward circle into a beneficial upward one.

I advised this woman to sing. Not sad songs but hymns of praise. To sing them out loud, not just hum, paying attention to the words. The issue in this woman's case was, in part, a spiritual one. Besides the fact that singing does wonders for the lungs and circulation, the words serve as a reminder of the wonders of creation that are all too easily forgotten in the face of hurt and disappointment. Asking the Lord's help in letting go of old habits and fears brings us to a strength greater than our own.

Nothing is really worth the slow dying that results from hanging on to old hopes and negative feelings, but human beings unfortunately seem to do so. In this we are like monkeys. In India and Africa, monkeys are caught in a simple kind of trap, a gourd filled with peanuts firmly anchored to a tree. There is a hole in the gourd large enough for the monkey's empty hand to slip through, but small enough that when the monkey tries to pull out his fist closed around the peanut, he cannot get it out through the hole. Rather than let go of the peanut, the monkey holds on and pulls and struggles until he is captured. I often tell patients this monkey story to help them in their struggle with old feelings. One day a man I was treating for depression

49

came in beaming. The first thing he said to me, in a triumphant booming voice was, "I dropped the peanut!"

Sometimes I suggest patients find a friend to talk out feelings with, rather than keeping them locked up inside. If no one is available, writing angers and hurts down on a piece of paper and then burning it can help to release the feelings.

4

Allergies

Allergies are very common in the United States. Millions of people are plagued with hay fever, post-nasal drip, sinus infections, skin allergies, food allergies, and now, environmental illness which has been described as an allergic reaction to the 20th Century. The people who suffer from environmental illness are nearly totally incapacitated by such things as the glue used to lay carpet, diesel exhaust, or perfume.

While recognizing the existence of pollen and the toxicity of many chemicals in our world today, Chinese medicine always asks: What is the condition of the patient's qi and blood? Is the middle burner able to absorb food? Collectively, these elements form the concept of righteous qi, a notion which Western physicians are now increasingly aware of as well. They call it immune competence. The basis of righteous qi is the condition of the spleen and stomach. When these two are able to digest and absorb the nourishment they take in, they create the qi which sustains strength internally and protects against external harm. (See Appendix E: Treatment of Auto-Immune Deficiency Syndrome — AIDS.)

The process of converting food into qi takes place in the middle burner, the collective functions of the spleen and stomach in Chinese physiology and of the liver, stomach, pancreas, and small intestine in Western physiology. It is no accident that this process is thought of as taking place in a "burner". What we know of metabolism in a Western sense indicates that digestion is a chemical process which takes place at a certain temperature for which we must maintain constant internal body heat. We are considered to be "warm blooded". The Chinese consider this process to be dependent on the fire in the body, and fire is the mother of earth. Only when fire is strong can the transformation of food into qi take place.

Much of the problem we see with allergies today is due to the fact that peoples' life-styles and habits do not support the production of righteous qi or the optimum functioning of the middle burner. With refrigeration and the custom of drinking iced drinks winter or summer, regardless of season, cold spleens are the rule, not the exception. Because of tight work schedules and long commute times, many people have formed the habits of skipping meals, especially breakfast, and working long hours despite exhaustion, without adequate nourishment or rest.

Both women and men fear being thought too heavy and attempt to keep themselves below their optimum weight by dieting, fasting, and avoiding calorie-rich foods such as rice. When they do eat, it may be fast food or cold, raw, simple food such as salad and as a consequence, they are malnourished.

The Chinese have long considered the qi which comes from rice and similar foods to be indispensable to life. We call it *gu qi*, the qi of grain. It is the qi which only grain can best provide. Meat too in small amounts, approximately 2 oz. at a time, and eggs are also necessary if a person is to maintain the yang qi necessary for survival in the busy world most of us must live in. Vegetarianism is only appropriate for those whose main activity is meditation and whose lives are lived in the shelter of a temple.

Lettuce and other raw vegetables contribute to both evil cold and dampness in the body. Such foods are cold because they are raw and because their character, the quality of the qi that they possess, is cold. Cucumbers and strawberries are especially cold in character. Oranges and other citrus fruits produce dampness. Both cold and dampness are detrimental to health.

Even some Oriental people have misunderstood why it was that the ancients warned against eating raw vegetables and drinking unboiled, cold water. After coming to the West, they thought that the danger of contamination was eliminated—in the East, human excrement is used as fertilizer. However, the old Chinese warning is still valid. Vegetables should be cooked and water boiled and drunk warm not only to kill disease-producing organisms but also to add warmth so that the body's fire does not have to exhaust itself by doing all the work.

The problem of cold food is an especially severe one for allergic patients, and is, indeed, in part, a cause of their condition. Cold food slows the metabolism and congests the qi. Heated food expands and promotes the flow of qi. Cold contracts and inhibits movement. Cold slows the liver, whose responsibility is to clean the blood. Acids accumulate in the blood and urine because the liver cannot adequately remove them from the blood. This accumulation of acid in the blood further inhibits the flow of qi and produces pain and stiffness throughout the body.

After a number of years of coldness affecting the spleen, stomach, and liver, the lungs too undergo pathological changes. Sneezing begins to occur frequently. And because of the damage to liver yin tears, redness, and itching occur in the eyes. When the lungs are absolutely cold, clear mucus runs down the throat, especially when the patient lies down. The mucus is produced by a cold spleen and the weakened lungs are unable to hold it back. This then results in post-nasal drip.

Once I was in an airplane where, as always, they served cold drinks. I usually refuse, but on this occasion, when the steward brought orange juice with ice, I took a glass. Immediately after drinking it, I started to sneeze and my eyes and nose ran for 4 hours. My sinuses were blocked and I felt just like I had a sinus allergy. Perhaps if I had not been so tired at that time, this one glass of cold juice would not have had so pronounced and sudden an effect, but I had been overworking for several months and my qi was depleted. The relationship between drinking the iced drink and the symptoms was obvious to me.

In this country, most people don't know how to make the connection between such symptoms and their intake of cold food and drink. Asthmatics, for instance, will often have to stop and breathe with their mouths open when drinking something cold too fast. The cold contracts the bronchi, while drinking something hot would help to expand them. Some Western doctors suggest ice cold drinks to stop wheezing, and, in some cases, this does provide temporary relief by tranquilizing bronchial spasms. But such relief is only short term, and rather than helping to get rid of the cause, it adds to it by generating cold phlegm which fills the lungs.

53

If allergy and asthma patients stop drinking cold juices and ice water and eating cold and raw foods at the same time that they receive treatment, they will recover much faster. One young man came for treatment for sinus allergy, hair loss, and fatigue. He received treatment twice a week for several months. He would feel better for a time and then his fatigue would return or his sinus condition would relapse. Finally, in exasperation, I asked him if he were still drinking or eating anything cold. He replied that, yes, he still had a large glass of cold orange juice first thing every morning. Once he stopped doing that, he began to recover as I had expected him to do in the first place. While acupuncture treatment is a powerful way to open the flow of qi and strengthen the body, wrong habits are also powerful in blocking qi and weakening the organs and can slow or inhibit the body's response to the needles.

The points used for allergy are the same as used for depression. Supplement *Zu San Li* (St 36) to strengthen the lungs. Drain *He Gu* (LI 4) and *Lie Que* (Lu 7) to get rid of the empty heat in the lungs. Although allergy is a cold condition, there is still empty heat in the lungs and also in the intestines as a result of stagnation and blockage of the qi of these 2 organs. These 2 points also regulate the lung qi. *Lie Que* (Lu 7) pulls up the qi and *He Gu* (LI 4) clears the lungs. Supplement *San Yin Jiao* (Sp 6) and drain *Qu Chi* (LI 11).

A. Asthma

I include asthma as a subcategory of allergy because it is simply a more severe response of the body to the same stimuli which cause other allergic reactions. Most asthma is due as much to cold in the stomach as it is due to cold weather. Even with severe cases, applying moxa in moxa pots to *Zhong Wan* (CV 12) and *Zu San Li* (St 36) will shorten the number of treatments. If the patient will cut back on tea and coffee, that will help the lungs also. Tea is cold in character even when it is drunk hot, and the body, already cold, does not need the extra cooling properties of the tea. Coffee is hot in character, but not in a beneficial way. The lungs are susceptible to extremes of either hot or cold. It is because of this sensitivity to temperature changes and the characteristic hot and cold qualities of foods that the lungs have been referred to in Chinese medicine as the delicate or tender organ.

54

Use the same needle combination as for allergy to strengthen the lungs and the spleen. *San Yin Jiao* (Sp 6) in this condition strengthens the kidney qi whose emptiness is at the root of chronic asthma. Diet is very important for asthmatics. If the patient has heat in the lungs as evidenced by yellow phlegm, drain *Zu San Li* (St 36 and do not use more moxa. (See Appendix F: Dietary Directions for Asthma/Emphysema)

B. Skin Allergies

In Chinese medicine, there is no concept identical to the Western concept of allergy. The condition here termed allergy is understood to be the body's response to poisons which have accumulated in the system. The Western disease hives includes many different kinds of skin eruptions which in Chinese medicine are categorized according to whether they are hot, *i.e.* red bumps, or cold, *i.e.*, white bumps.

Needling alone, even using these powerful points, does not give lasting results in such skin conditions, although patients will calm down immediately and fall asleep peacefully on the table, the itching relieved for a short time. In addition to needles, I use *Fu Zi Li Zhong Wan*, an herbal formula with Radix Praeparatus Aconiti Carmichaeli (*Fu Zi*), a very warming herb, to regulate and warm the center. *Li Zhong Wan* with Cortex Cinnamomi (*Rou Gui*) will work also.

Urticaria or skin on which raised, red, itching welts appear after slight scratching, is due to too much false heat and sugar in the blood. In children, it is due to sweets, and in adults to alcohol and/or sweets. Drain *Zu San Li* (St 36) to clear heat from the heart by draining the son.

5

Nervousness & Emotional Disturbances

The relationship of righteous qi to emotional stability and the ability to handle stress has already been mentioned. The following cases illustrate this connection.

A. Self-pity & Over-reaction

A young man 25 years old came to me. He was very artistic and musical and had great inner pride and sensitivity. He did not say much, but I knew that when he was 19 he had taken a test to enter art school and had been turned down. His friend, who had failed in school, passed the test and was accepted. The boy felt that his friend could only have gotten in by favoritism, not ability. In response to his anger and disappointment, he refused to draw, play piano, sleep, eat, or talk. The youngest and only boy in a family with 4 older sisters who always tried to help him, he was very spoiled and accustomed to getting his own way. He refused to try the examination again.

Recently, he had gotten up in the middle of the night and had broken the television. The reason he gave was that 2 of his sisters had argued over which channel to watch. He overheard this argument and became angry. He held in his feelings until midnight when he destroyed the set. Though he had continued going to work, he could not study. On the job, he felt that his co-workers were making fun of him and giving him the dirty work to do. Feeling abused and sorry for himself, he quarreled with them and the firm let him go. After he lost his job, his mother brought him in to see me.

I told him about my own life as the only girl with 6 brothers. My self-pity and anger were so great that I often had a stomachache or a headache. I would pout and go 2 or more days without eating if I felt myself mistreated. My mother, recognizing what was going on, ignored me. Finally I realized that my stomachache was not real, that I used it when I wanted to get attention from my family who were all too busy with their own affairs. When I saw that my pain was not getting me what I wanted, I said to myself, "I am strong, I can work and make happen what I want to have happen." The boy laughed as I described by self-pity and my pain. He recognized himself in my story.

I gave him *Zu San Li* (St 36), *He Gu* (LI 4), and *Lie Que* (Lu 7), and because he was thin with small, weak muscles, I also used *San Yin Jiao* (Sp 6) and *Qu Chi* (LI 11). After the second treatment, the boy stopped boasting loudly that he could do everything. After the fourth treatment, he became very calm. His sleeping habits became regular. Instead of staying up late into the night, he slept early and got up early to draw, work in the garden, and practice his music. The whole family noticed the changes. After that, I went on vacation and did not treat him further as he had no more outbreaks and was headed in a positive direction.

B. Nervousness

A young woman came to my office. She was a school teacher who had worked with teenagers for 5 years. She loved her work, but the tension of having to deal with adolescent tricks made her uneasy and irritable. She had young children of her own, and, when she was upset at school she could not tolerate their demands when she got home. She had also been having increasing difficulty falling asleep.

During her vacation, she came up from Los Angeles for treatment. Her pulse was tight and she was very tired. I gave her *Zu San Li* (St 36), *He Gu* (LI 4), and *Lie Que* (Lu 7) and the sleeping point on the bottom of the foot near the heel. (See Appendix D for illustrations of extra points.)

As soon as I applied the needles, she sighed, closed her eyes, and dozed off. The second day when she came in, she was joyful, chatting about how she felt like dancing. She was a different woman from the exhausted, harried person who had come to my office the day before. I gave her the name of an acupuncturist in L.A., so she could continue treatments at home.

C. Biting Fingernails

Case 1

A woman was married to a successful business man. She was very beautiful and had nothing which she had to do. They had no children, lived in a large house which she had servants keep immaculate, and she entertained her husband in the evenings with superb dinners. But she was extremely nervous. No one, including herself, knew why. She came to me because she wanted a face lift, which I do not do, as there are so many ill people who need my time and energy more than those who simply want to look younger. About to tell her this and refuse her, I noticed that all 10 of her fingernails were bitten to the quick. She had not been able to allow them to grow a millimeter for 6 years. If she didn't bite them they itched until she couldn't stand it, she said.

The nails are related to the liver. When they become soft, this indicates a weakness in the liver. When they itch and biting calms them, the spleen and kidneys are implicated also. The liver cannot control the spleen, the spleen overcontrols the kidneys, and thus the person is nervous and anxious.

One treatment with *Zu San Li* (St 36), *He Gu* (LI 4), and *Lie Que* (Lu 7) stopped the itching. Even though these point do not directly deal with the liver, supplementing the stomach and nourishing the lungs both nourishes and controls the kidneys. When the kidneys are strong, they can nourish the liver, their son, and the nails will then flourish. Soon the woman's nails grew long and beautiful, and, while this is not important in itself, her increased calmness was a benefit to her and to all who knew her.

Case 2

A 16 year old school girl with no apparent great pressures in her life came in for treatment to stop biting her nails. It is possible that in some cases, there is no external source of tension. The feeling can be generated

59

internally. The problem then is on the level of the channels and not the organs, and treatment calms the nerves quickly. This girl only needed 2 treatments. If the patient has many difficult problems to resolve in their life, more treatments are needed to strengthen the organs' ability to withstand the ongoing pressures.

Case 3

One woman had fingernails so sensitive that if she scratched her head, she created static electricity and her fourth finger would experience a strong shock. The fourth finger belongs to the triple heater channel and relates to emotions. This woman had had many problems with her 20 year old son, and, while her head did not itch, she was continually scratching it and getting shocked.

Sometimes when people come to me with something like this, I can only shake may head and say, "The human body does funny things!" Fortunately, even such strange problems can be solved by a careful application of Chinese acupuncture theory. Strong emotion, overjoy or extreme sadness or, in her case, worry and anger, can imbalance the qi in the channels. Using my formula calmed the woman and corrected this imbalance. The electrical sensitivity in her fourth finger went away.

(See Appendix G, Mental Degeneration Beginning with a Tight Stomach, for the progressive stages of emotional disturbance.)

6

Weight Loss

Some overweight people eat excessively and so gain weight. Others eat little and still they become heavier. Acupuncture treatment is different for these 2 types.

A. Excessive Eating

For those who eat excessively and are always hungry, use the hunger points on the ear, inserting them in the following order: Heart/Thyroid point, Internal Secretion, Hunger Point, Kidney, Sympathetic, and *Shen Men*. (See Appendix D for locations of points.) *Shen Men* is the most painful, so it is needled last. Because it is the most likely to bleed, it should also be removed last and then covered with cotton if need be.

Imbalances known as thyroid problems in Western medicine are related to the heart in Chinese medicine. Full fire effects earth. Food is burned too rapidly and the person feels hungry soon after eating, needing more food to maintain their blood sugar level. Because earth is imbalanced, it is unable to perform its function of moving water throughout the body, and dampness accumulates. It is this dampness which makes the person swollen, large, and heavy.

Ordinarily when treating digestive disturbances, we want the person to be able to absorb food better. In this case, however, we want the person to eliminate water. Therefore, drain *Zu San Li* (St 36) and *San Yin Jiao* (Sp 6) and supplement *He Gu* (LI 4), *Qu Chi* (LI 11), and *Lie Que* (Lu 7) to increase urination. The ear points mentioned above eliminate cravings, adjust the internal secretions, and calm the spirit, while the body points strengthen the functioning of the organs involved. The patient must also deal with his or her habits of eating frequently and excessively in response to stress and upset.

B. Heavy People Who Do Not Overeat

Heavy people who do not eat much but still gain weight also have water retention in the cells of their bodies due to spleen dampness. The swelling they experience has a different character from that of the previous type of overweight person. In this instance, when the body is pressed with the finger, there is no pitting. The finger leaves no dent after pressing. Whereas the previous type was solidly waterlogged, this type is wet and puffy in an empty kind of way. There is no real energy in the cells. Most of these people eat lots of raw salads and drink cold drinks. They get no real nourishment from their diets. Although they eat less and less, they get larger and emptier due to the empty spleen's inability to transport and transform water dampness.

Treatment is to nourish the blood and boost the qi. As true qi is supplied to the cells, the wetness is driven out. The person begins to shrink back to normal size. To rid the body of excess wetness, *Zu San Li* (St 36), and *San Yin Jiao* (Sp 6), must be drained; *He Gu* (LI 4), *Qu Chi* (LI 11), and *Lie Que* (Lu 7) must be supplemented. Then immediately *Zu San Li* (St 36), *San Yin Jiao* (Sp 6), must be supplemented, and *He Gu* (LI 4), *Qu Chi* (LI 11), and *Lie Que* (Lu 7) drained. Do the 9's first, then the 6's on the metal channels, and the 6's first, then the 9's on earth points. This removes the excess wetness and also strengthens the weakness. While the underlying problem is one of deficiency and emptiness, it is important to remove the accumulated dampness to make room for the true qi to enter. However, unless there is supplementation provided also, the person cannot regain strength, and, in fact, will feel weaker. Drainage treatments deplete some of the true qi as well as dispersing false qi or evil fullness.

Dietary changes are imperative for strength to be regained and weight to be lost. The patient needs to eat lots of white rice, cooked vegetables, a little lean meat, and fermented soy products. Fish should be cooked with ginger, as without the ginger to warm it, it is too cold in character. Beef should be avoided, as it tends to make muscles larger. Shellfish is also too cold.

C. Anorexia & Bulimia

Often young women are afraid to gain weight and they starve themselves. Hunger damages the spleen leaving the patient unable to eat, even if they wanted to. When the stomach qi is empty, the patient becomes afraid of crowds. She dislikes noise and must eat alone, afraid people will look at her. This is the opposite of the stomach excess type of madness where one runs naked through the streets. (This is further described in Appendix G.)

Supplementation of *Zu San Li* (St 36), *San Yin Jiao* (Sp 6), and drainage of *He Gu* (LI 4), *Qu Chi* (LI 11), and *Lie Que* (Lu 7) strengthens and reopens the digestion. The hunger points on the ear are also appropriate here because they adjust the metabolism. If it is too low, they increase it. If it is hyperactive, they slow it down. If the patient vomits whenever she eats, add *Nei Guan* (Per 6) and/or bleed *Feng Fu* (GV 16).

8

Hypoglycemia, Hyperglycemia, & Diabetes

Both hypoglycemia and hyperglycemia or diabetes are problems of internal secretion imbalance. Chinese medicine sees hypo and hyperglycemia as two ends of the spectrum in the same disease. In hypoglycemia, the internal secretion system responds with too much insulin, thus pulling sugar out of the blood rapidly. In diabetes, the internal secretion system has become exhausted and is unable to supply enough insulin. Hence too much sugar remains in the blood. Both conditions are a problem of damage to earth or the spleen and stomach.

The body, out of balance, craves the sweet taste. Too little sweet leaves the spleen weak, too much drains it. This craving is usually "satisfied" by candy, pastries, soft drinks made with sugar, a refined, super-concentrated extract far different from its original sources. As such, sugar is a potent yang substance, so strong that it is toxic to the body. It generates excessive heat of a false kind and leads to yin emptiness.

Treatment in this case does not use *Zu San Li* (St 36) which one would have expected, but rather 3 points on the spleen channel. These points are so potent they have come to be called the 3 Emperors. They are *San Yin Jiao* (Sp 6), *Lou Gu* (Sp 7), and a third point 1½ inches below *Yin Ling Quan* (Sp 9) called *Shen Guan* or Kidney Gate. All 3 are supplemented.

Zu San Li (St 36) can be used, but these 3 points work much better. Diabetes is a yang full, yin empty condition. Therefore using the spleen or the yin earth channel has a stronger effect.

Sweet Cravings

Many people, both overweight and thin, are plagued by cravings for sweets. This is an internal secretion problem, and the Hunger Points already mentioned are very effective when used 3–5 days in a row. The Hunger Point itself is near (SI 19). The Heart/Thyroid point is really neither heart or thyroid in Chinese medicine. It is called the Heart Secretion or Heart Organ point (*Xin Zang Dian*). The formula also includes Kidney, *Shen Men*, and Sympathetic points. This makes this formula useful for people who cannot sleep, have no appetite, and/or swollen arms and legs as well.

These problems, excessive or no appetite, excessive heaviness or thinness, lethargy or over-excitement, are related to what Western physicians think of as hyper and hypothyroidism. Ear points regulate all the glands in the brain which control hormonal and enzymatic activity throughout the body. Salt cravings are also reflective of internal secretion imbalance and the same points are used.

9

Upper Respiratory Tract Problems

A. Colds, Flu, Bronchitis & Sore Throat

As mentioned in Section 1, *He Gu* (LI 4) and *Qu Chi* (LI 11) scatter wind from the surface of the body. They clear upper burner heat and open the orifices and senses of the head. *Lie Que* (Lu 7) transforms phlegm and moistens dry throat. In addition to its ability to supplement the lungs by strengthening earth, *Zu San Li* (St 36) can break fever by inducing perspiration, and it also increases the white blood cell count. For these reasons, I use these points at the first sign of a cold or the flu.

If there is a bad cough with yellow-green phlegm, I drain *Chi Ze* (Lu 5), the water point. This is based on draining the son to drain heat in the mother. If the cough is dry and the throat scratchy, have the patient fry an egg in 2–3 Tb. roasted sesame oil until the yolk is hard and then eat the egg. *Nin Jiom Pei Pa Kao*, Loquat Cough Syrup, is very good for cough with an oncoming cold and *Chuan Bei Mu,* Fritillaria Extract is helpful for deep, severe cough. (Also see Appendix H, Winter Pear and Rock Sugar for Reducing Phlegm.)

For sore throat, in addition to needling the main points, bleeding *Shao Shang* (Lu 11) and *Shang Yang* (LI 1) gives immediate relief if treated early enough or while the disease is still in the channels.

B. Pneumonia

The signs of pneumonia are fever, thick yellow or green phlegm, and the nostrils flaring in and out when the patient breathes. The color of the phlegm indicates that lung tissue is dying and the situation is very serious. Begin treating immediately using very strong stimulation. Supplement *Zu San Li* (St 36) and *San Yin Jiao* (Sp 6) thus increasing earth to generate metal. Drain *He Gu* (LI 4), *Qu Chi* (LI 11), and *Lie Que* (Lu 7) to clear the evil heat. This will eliminate the phlegm rapidly. If the onset is very acute, bleed *Shao Shang* (Lu 11), *Shang Yang* (LI 1), and *Chi Ze* (Lu 5) to reduce the sucking air quality of the breathing. Again, this treatment is only effective at the very beginning while the heat is still in the channel. After that, the disease is in the organ and bleeding the channels will have no effect.

Acupuncture treatment for pneumonia should be relied on only when it is possible to stay with the patient and give treatment every 6 hours, night and day. If such intensive treatment is not possible, do not delay in sending the patient to the hospital.

C. Recovering from Respiratory Infection

I often see people who were hospitalized for pneumonia. One to several months later, they are still exhausted and have recovered little of their former strength and vitality. Using *Zu San Li* (St 36), *San Yin Jiao* (Sp 6), *He Gu* (LI 4), *Qu Chi* (LI 11), and *Lie Que* (Lu 7) helps to restore their qi very quickly.

If the patient recovering from severe respiratory infection is weak or elderly, it is of vital importance that they be given nourishing food whether they have been treated with antibiotics or acupuncture. Especially after antibiotics, there is the possibility that a lingering low-grade fever will remain even though the medication was powerful enough to knock out the bacteria. It is important to realize that this type of fever is not caused by bacteria or full heat evil but is due to emptiness. Proper nourishment for the patient is the key to recovery. For this type of weak, deficient patient, a good strong broth of game hen with egg noodles can make all the difference. (See Appendix I, Not All Fever is Caused by Infection.)

D. Lung Collapse

A 55 year old woman, whose husband had been dead for a year, grieved constantly. Even after this length of time, she still wept uncontrollably whenever she thought of his death. She came infrequently, never really committing herself to treatment. I told her that she would soon follow her husband if she continued to lose so much qi grieving and that, by clinging to his memory, she would interfere with what he needed to do in the next life. One day she came in with excruciating pain. Her doctor had taken x-rays which indicated that her lung had collapsed. From Chinese theory we can understand what happened to her. Constant grieving and worry weakened her lung qi and damaged her spleen. No longer able to withstand the gravity of the earth and life, her lung had collapsed. I tried several other treatments to relieve the pain with no result. Therefore, I decided to treat the source, returning to my formula. The change was immediate and profound. She gave a sigh and the gasping, crying sound which had accompanied her every inhale ceased. When she left the office, she was relatively free from pain. She had 8 treatments, following which an x-ray showed that her lung had re-expanded. I have had a number of cases in which acupuncture restoration of the lung has been verified by x-ray.

A patient such as this may continue to experience similar symptoms as long as she holds on to the feelings that weaken her. Some patients come for a few treatments and experience an emotional release as well as a physical one. They feel themselves cured, and I may not see them again for another 10 years, during which time they are happy and productive. Other patients are unwilling to let go of whatever it is that makes them sick. These people need to come for many more treatments, enough to make a substantial difference in the qi of the lung and spleen organs. When the organs are stronger, it is much easier to move beyond memories and grief. Inability to stop grieving is both a symptom of weakness and one of its causes. Some part of this woman held on to both her grief and her illness so that she would never follow through on a course of treatment even though she knew it would help her.

69

When a patient holds onto problems like this, there is little even the most astute acupuncturist can do, except to recognize the choice the patient is making. I never agree to such a choice myself, and I won't give up even when the patient has. As long as someone comes, I will treat them, knowing that it is always possible to choose life. I may tell a story from my own experience, of the time when I was close to death and had to let go to a purpose greater than my own in order to regain my health and return to work. It is important to communicate to my patients, from a very deep place inside myself, that such healing is possible. I know it is, for I have experienced it.

Therapeutic Uses of
Zu San Li (St 36) Alone

There are a number of conditions which can be treated by using *Zu San Li* (St 36) alone. Nausea is a function of the qi of the stomach rising when it should go down. *Zu San Li* (St 36) lowers it. Because the stomach earth is the son of heart fire, *Zu San Li* (St 36) can be used to treat heart problems. And because the stomach channel runs along the mammillary line, *Zu San Li* (St 36) can also be used for problems of the breast.

Nausea & Gagging

Case 1

A man, 72 years of age, came to see me for nausea. He'd had dentures for 4 years before his wife died. After her death he became very down-hearted, and in the following 2 years he developed trouble wearing his dentures. Whenever he put them in his mouth, he gagged and felt nauseous. After he met a woman whom he wanted to marry, he came to see me. Treatment with *Zu San Li* (St 36) calmed him and restored the supply of oxygen to his brain. Soon he was able to smile at his new bride with his dentures in.

Case 2

A 16 year old boy was very busy. He was a leader in his class, he enjoyed literature, played sports, and had a job. Suddenly, whenever he ate, he found himself vomiting up his food. This reaction occurred whenever food reached his throat. Though he was hungry, he could not eat and had lost weight. I gave him *Zu San Li* (St 36) plus *Nei Guan* (Per 6) and the next day he ate 4 pieces of toast, 2 eggs, and a glass of milk for breakfast. That was the only treatment necessary.

Pallor

When the face is pale, we know that the patient's heart qi is weak and that the qi is unable to rise to the face. Also the blood is empty. Supplementing *Zu San Li* (St 36) adjusts the heart, and, after stimulation, you will see the face infused with a vibrant rosy color.

Heart Problems

If the heart rate is too slow, treat the liver (mother) to supplement the heart (son) since wood generates fire. *Xing Jian* (Liv 2) and *Tai Chong* (Liv 3) have the most powerful effect on the heart. They are near the great toe which is an important part of their potency.

For excessively rapid heart beat, drain the son or stomach. *Zu San Li* (St 36) may be used or 2 special points on the stomach channel called Four Flower Middle. These points are located 4 and 5 *cun* below *Zu San Li* (St 36). The point 6 *cun* down is *Tiao Kou* (St 38) and should be drained by inserting the needles very deep, 2–3 inches, and not manipulating them. Leave then in for 45 minutes and then, just prior to withdrawal, supplement. These points control the kidneys, helping to rebalance the heart and kidneys. This is another instance of the use of earth channel points to rebalance fire and water.

Hypertension

High blood pressure can best be thought of in terms of a husband and wife who are not getting along. When they are not on good terms, the wife does not want to stay at home, so she leaves. When the husband comes home tired from work and finds the home cold and empty, he too leaves and goes to the bar where he drinks and finds other men to joke or argue with.

In the body, it is the same. If there is too much yang activity, yin is decreased. When yin becomes empty and deficient, there is nothing to which the yang can anchor and it goes out all the more. This energetic pattern results in symptoms which are called hypertension in Western terminology and liver yang rising in Chinese terms. We distinguish between full yang and yin empty types. Empty, deficient types are more due to overwork, exhaustion, working night shifts, lack of sleep, and coldness. Yang types are also a response to overwork, but generally the patient has used stimulants, such as spicy food, cigarettes, coffee, alcohol, chocolate, or caffeinated soft drinks to keep their flagging energy going. The accumulated toxins from all these heating, yang substances and from running on empty create a condition of fullness. High blood pressure may also be caused by medicines, such as prednisone, or from diets high in rich and fatty foods which cause cholesterol deposits and hardening of the arteries.

Generally, when only the upper number which represents the systolic pressure is high, the condition is due to a plethora of yang. When the lower number representing the diastolic pressure is high, the condition is due to emptiness of yin. When both are high, there is both too much yang and insufficient yin.

Even in the case of yang fullness, it can easily be seen that the root of the problem is still one of emptiness of yin qi. In the treatment of either type of hypertension, rather than draining yang, it is better to supplement yin, or true yin energy. *Zu San Li* (St 36), though on a yang channel, supplements spleen yin as well as strengthening true yang. When yin is strengthened, the yang automatically returns home to its lower source. The fullness is reduced, the yang that has been misspent is restored, and it, in turn, can protect the yin, for true and harmonious yang protects and generates yin.

Therefore, for hypertension, supplement *Zu San Li* (St 36). If there is a plethora of evil yang, as in toxic residues from stimulants or excessive emotions and exhaustion, and the upper and lower readings are both too high, also bleed the back along the bladder channel and cup to draw out the dark, stagnant blood. Together these treatments will bring pressure down instantaneously as they supplement both true yin and true yang and drain excess yang. This achieves more lasting results than treatment which simply

73

attempt to drain the effulgent yang. Unless the true yin and true yang are strengthened, draining techniques give only temporary relief. Supplementing *Zu San Li* (St 36) with *Guan Yuan* (CV 4) and *Qi Hai* (CV 6) works amazingly quickly and powerfully. It can drop the reading 20 or more points immediately. The patient typically falls asleep on the treatment table and wakes feeling refreshed.

Herbs are especially important in this case. Again, *Fu Zi Li Zhong Wan* is the formula I use. Because it regulates the center, it is able to balance yin and yang, supplying more yin through supplementing true yang rather than draining the false or effulgent yang.

Breast Pain

This condition is a result of the interplay between hormones and anxiety. For many women, there is a dark cloud around or just behind them, especially as they near the ages of 60 or 70. They fear cancer of their reproductive organs and are anxious and nervous. Most of these women have made a lifelong habit of these emotions. There is always one reason or another to worry. This internal tension imbalances the internal secretion system which regulates the reproductive system. This emotional anxiety translates into physical tightness and qi congestion along the channels. When emotions lead the liver qi to congest and wood to overcontrol earth, pain along the course of the stomach channel which goes through the center of the breasts may occur.

Treating *Zu San Li* (St 36) with a special technique which uses both draining (*xie fa*) and supplementing (*bu fa*) alternated repeatedly is an excellent way to open the stomach channel. However, to keep the qi flowing through the channels, the tension must be resolved and lifelong habits of worrying and expecting the worst must be addressed.

One woman I treated in Sweden had had breast pain for 6 or 7 years. Her husband had died, leaving her with much property to manage. Her son would not accept any responsibility for this fortune or its management, and she was angry with him and very worried. After the first treatment using the above mentioned technique on *Zu San Li* (St 36), her pain was gone, but 2 days later it came back. I treated her for 10 days and the pain left and did not return.

This kind of breast pain is different from pain due to engorged breasts during nursing or from the pain which comes just before or during the menstrual period. These are cases of full qi in the stomach channel. Simply draining *Zu San Li* (St 36) will relieve the premenstrual distention and fullness. If the woman is a new mother with too much milk congested in her breasts, she should eat less chicken broth and other extra-nourishing foods. (In China, women are given rich broths, large quantities of eggs, etc. after delivery to help them regain their strength). Draining *He Gu* (LI 4) and *Lie Que* (Lu 7) or metal, earth's son, relieves the pain.

Worms

In children especially, roundworms stay in the intestines where it is warm and rich in nutrients. The worms prefer sluggish intestines with weak peristalsis so they can rest there comfortably. Over time, they accumulate and can block the movement of stool through the bowels. Children lose weight and their bellies become enlarged. Their faces become greenish and there may be pale patches on the stomach channel area of the cheeks. They become increasingly malnourished and have more and more abdominal pain.

In this case draining *Zu San Li* (St 36) increases peristalsis and nourishes the large intestine. When movement increases in the intestines, it feels to the worms like an earthquake and they move away, no longer feeling safe. They come out in the stool, in severe cases by the hundreds. Many times, soon after the needles are applied, I must remove them so the child can run to the rest room to begin the process.

The Special Properties of *Zu San Li* (St 36)

These powerful applications of *Zu San Li* (St 36) lead us to a discussion of its powerful effect of the body. In Chinese, it is called *Zu San Li*. This is directly translated as Foot Three Miles or Three Measures. Various interpretations are given for this name. Because it is 3 inches below the knee, it is called Three Measures. It is also said that needling it will enable a totally exhausted person to walk another 3 miles.

It has also been written of this point that needling it powerfully will "chase evil from the 4 limbs to a distance 3 miles away". Sending evil qi out through the toes is what I remember when I used *Zu San Li* (St 36), another reason why I feel it is very important for the stimulation to go all the way down to and out the toes. One of my patients is convinced that I send the qi not only out the toes but through the wall on the other side of the treatment room!

When giving strong stimulation, the idea is to induce qi to go where it is needed by searching for and directing it. *Huan Tiao* (GB 30) is another point where this technique is especially used. Probe in the eight directions. Down to the center makes 9—drawing and pulling with the needle until the qi goes to the toe. Such strong stimulation can only be given in an area of the body which is large and well-muscled. It is not possible between bones or through small foramina. Also avoid strong stimulation on very weak patients or they may faint. Patients with heart disease should also not receive strong stimulation.

The stomach channel begins on the head and travels to the chest. From the chest, it goes to the navel. From there, it travels down the leg and foot to the earth. Draining *Zu San Li* (St 36) calms the liver and brings evil qi down and out the body through the intestines. In ancient texts it is mentioned that supplementing *Zu San Li* (St 36) can stop long term loose stools, but I prefer to use *Nei Ting* (St 44) and *Xian Gu* (St 43), as mentioned previously.

The ancients also refer to its powerful effect on mental patients, particularly those of the manic type who run naked through the streets singing songs. This is a full yang type of madness. The boy who broke the TV set was perhaps beginning to experience this type of disturbance.

It is of vital importance to use the proper type of stimulation on *Zu San Li* (St 36). When catching cold, in the beginning stage when the upper body is hot and the lower part is cold, supplement *Zu San Li* (St 36) to increase lung qi to fight off external evils while draining *He Gu* (LI 4) and *Lie Que* (Lu 7). If the stimulation which you give *Zu San Li* (St 36) drains it, the patient will become sicker because you have knocked out the lung qi and with it the *wei* or protective qi.

Fortunately with needles, you can quickly correct the treatment and reestablish the lung qi. Unlike herbs and moxa, substances which, having gone into the body, will stay there whether they are appropriate or not, needle treatments can easily be reversed as they work on the qi of the body directly. The key to knowing if your technique is correct is to watch the patient's responses carefully. The face should become gently flushed and warm, the breathing should slow and deepen, and the person should relax or fall asleep. If the face pales, the person experiences coldness, tightness, restlessness, and the respiration becomes more shallow and rapid, the treatment has had the wrong effect. The technique was wrong and must be reversed.

For the elderly or the chronically ill, supplementation (and moxa) of *Zu San Li* (St 36) and drainage of *He Gu* (LI 4) (no moxa) can only strengthen. I find that these points work much the same as the herbs Radix Panacis Ginseng (*Ren Shen*), Rhizoma Atractylodis Macrocephalae (*Bai Zhu*), and Cortex Cinnamomi (*Rou Gui*) which together strengthen the upper, middle, and lower energy centers of the body: the chest qi, the middle burner, and the *ming men* or life gate. The power of these points in contributing to health and long life cannot be over-emphasized.

Treating Children

An important point to remember with *Zu San Li* (St 36) is that for young people under 20 years of age, frequent moxa applied to this point may throw the body's temperature regulating mechanism out of balance. There is one interesting case recorded in the Chinese medical literature of a young man under 20 who received moxa 100 times on *Zu San Li* (St 36). His sensitivity to the world was entirely changed. On cold days, he wore light clothing and wanted cold food and drinks. The cold drinks seemed to him to be too hot, so he blew on them to cool them off. On hot days, he wore heavy garments and wanted hot food and drinks. Ever since, moxa for young people has been approached with caution.

In addition, it has been observed that children treated with excessive moxibustion may not grow or may grow too fast. This is because the moxa produces strong changes in the body. While it is still growing, the body is too sensitive to such intense stimulation.

Because of this sensitivity in growing children, we treat them carefully. The safest treatment is to bleed the Four Seams or *Si Feng* (M-UE-9) to rebalance the body. These points are on the pericardium, heart, triple heater, small and large intestine channels. Those channels which are imbalanced will have a clear, yellowish lymph-like fluid which comes out first when they are squeezed. Then blood will come out. When the lymph is removed, the appetite returns and the child feels better. If the child has been eating wrong, there will be more lymph than blood from the index finger. If the problem is more due to the child's inner emotions, the fourth finger will have more lymph. While if they take in the stresses of those around them, the third finger will have more lymph. Lymph from the fifth finger indicates imbalance in the heart.

I use these points for children who have poor digestion and bowel movements, for asthma, and every 6 months for children who are growing too slowly. It is especially useful for children who eat a lot but stay skinny. After treatment, the child may shoot up several inches or begin to gain weight. For little ones who have big bellies with many visible blood vessels, bleed the *Si Feng* (M-UE-9) and then supplement *Zu San Li* (St 36) and drain *He Gu* (LI 4).

10

Technique & Intention: Getting Patients Well

People ask me, "Do you teach everything you know or do you keep some techniques secret?" I have no hesitation to answer, "I hide nothing." To practice acupuncture, you must be certain of your intention, your purpose in doing so. It can be done for fame or wealth, to cure or to kill. If the intention is wrong, if you are concentrating on earning money, treating fewer patients and charging higher fees, doing little for much profit, you may get some results from your treatments or you may not.

Perhaps you make great claims in print and your name becomes well known, or you hate a patient, or for political reasons you put the needle just a little deeper, into the liver, perhaps. The person dies later without anyone knowing what happened. Wealth, power, fame, revenge—all these are possible.

But if you intend to cure, you use all your might to treat patients. You study, you concentrate, you learn all you can. Then when you are with your patients, the best of your knowledge and technique comes to you. Supplementation or drainage, you have a sure feeling what is called for. Even today, after so many years of having a heavy patient load, I sometimes still need to take a longer time with some patients, to change points, to dig deeper into my knowledge, to take a second look at who they are in order to relieve their distress. I want patients to leave my office feeling better. I do not rush them in and out without caring how they are and whether their condition has really been improved.

I have a good feeling towards the patients. The intention I have for them to get well travels, as a wave travels on the sea, from me to them through the needles and through my voice and eyes and hands. I use my qi very consciously in a special way to do this.

The needle technique I use is a part of this intention. Paying attention is the most important thing. Where you put the needle is also very important. You must put it in the right place. Insert it slowly and observe. Does the muscle hold the needle tight? If so, drain. Does the muscle feel like tofu, loose and limp? If so, supplement until the qi comes. You do not supplement always in exactly the same place, but pull the needle up and put it down at a slightly different angle, exploring, probing for the qi. When you feel the qi engage the needle, you are in just the right place. If the qi comes fast, drain, then supplement. If the qi comes slowly, supplement, then drain. All the time that you are reading the responses of the qi to the needle, you are also feeling your intention to make the person well with what you are doing. If your mind goes somewhere else, to food or your husband or paying the bills or advertising, you cannot concentrate on the technique.

I need have no secrets. Often, even when I tell someone how to use the needles, they do not get it. Their intention is not right or it is not strong enough or focused in the right way. Very few people know how to direct their intention.

This intention for the patient to get well travels like an electric wave to the person being needled. It is all my qi marshalled to meet their own intention to get well. Some patients do not have this intention themselves, they are so used to being sick. Perhaps they are avoiding some of life's responsibilities, or they are afraid of the world, or someone's care of them in their illness feels to them like love. They do not want to lose the nurturance and so they hold on to the illness as well. Or they simply do not believe they can get well and have given up. Many peoples' intentions are weak and unfocused and they lack knowledge of how to take care of themselves.

My intention for my patients to get well must awaken their own will and desire for recovery. If they can feel better after one treatment, they will have something real to trust, to base their hope on. Many of them have been sick for a long time. They have been to many doctors, chiropractors, and other acupuncturists, and I am a last resort. They may have come from far away. I come far to meet them.

There are many people practicing acupuncture now. Of all the important things they need to learn, the most important is how to give their whole-hearted attention to the patient's recovery.

Appendix A: The Five Transport Points

Channel	Well	Gushing	Transporting	Traversing	Uniting
Lung	Shao Shang (Lu 11)	Yu Ji (Lu 10)	Tai Yuan (Lu 9)	Jing Qu (Lu 8)	Chi Ze (Lu 5)
Pericardium	Zhong Chong (Per 9)	Lao Gong (Per 8)	Da Ling (Per 7)	Jian Shi (Per 5)	Qu Ze (Per 3)
Heart	Shao Chong (Ht 9)	Shao Fu (Ht 8)	Shen Men (Ht 7)	Ling Dao (Ht 4)	Shao Hai (Ht 3)
Spleen	Yin Bai (Sp 1)	Da Du (Sp 2)	Tai Bai (Sp 3)	Shang Qiu (Sp 5)	Yin Ling Quan (Sp 9)
Liver	Da Dun (Liv 1)	Xing Jian (Liv 2)	Tai Chong (Liv 3)	Zhong Feng (Liv 4)	Qu Quan (Liv 8)
Kidney	Yong Quan (Ki 1)	Ran Gu (Ki 2)	Tai Xi (Ki 3)	Fu Liu (Ki 7)	Yin Gu (Ki 10)
Large Intestine	Shang Yang (LI 1)	Er Jian (LI 2)	San Jian (LI 3)	Yang Xi (LI 5)	Qu Chi (LI 11)
Triple Heater	Guan Chong (TH 1)	Ye Men (TH 2)	Zhong Zhu (TH 3)	Zhi Gou (TH 6)	Tian Jing (TH 10)
Small Intestine	Shao Ze (SI 1)	Qian Gu (SI 2)	Hou Xi (SI 3)	Yang Gu (SI 5)	Xiao Hai (SI 8)
Stomach	Li Dui (St 45)	Nei Ting (St 44)	Xian Gu (St 43)	Jie Xi (St 41)	Zu San Li (St 36)
Gallbladder	Qiao Yin (GB 44)	Xia Xi (GB 43)	Zu Lin Qi (GB 41)	Yang Fu (GB 38)	Yang Ling Quan (GB-34)
Bladder	Zhi Yin (Bl 67)	Tong Gu (Bl 66)	Shu Gu (Bl 65)	Kun Lun (Bl 60)	Wei Zhong (Bl 40)

Appendix B

The Heart & Kidney in Traditional Chinese Medicine

The heart in traditional Chinese medicine is not the muscles or the valves of the anatomical heart. Rather, it is a certain aspect of human energy which the Chinese consider to be the king or ruler of human character. The heart houses the spirit and its qi underlies thought and intelligence, vitality and alertness, and the ability to speak clearly. For instance, it is said that the heart opens into the tongue. The heart also rules the blood, the blood vessels, and the pulse.

When functioning properly, it is the heart qi which maintains the person's inner balance in the face of external stress, criticism and praise, and the realization or thwarting of desire. The desire to obtain material possessions and success is one manifestation of its functioning, and when its qi is too strong, obsession, repetitive thoughts, inability to experience satisfaction, and madness may result.

Heart qi should go down to warm the feet and hands, and the cheeks should be rosy. If the cheeks are pale, we know that the heart qi is weak. If the extremities are cold, the heart may be weak or its qi may be flushing up to the head to be caught up in excessive and restive thinking with little qi directed to the rest of the body. Bright red cheeks, cold extremities, rapid pulse, disturbing thoughts, nervousness, and insomnia are signs of heart fire controlling the brain. This condition should never be treated by draining the heart directly. In fact, the heart channel should rarely be used. While no problem may be obvious at the time of treatment, harm may arise in the future. The pericardium channel can be used instead to regulate the heart, but more important is the interaction of the heart and kidneys.

While heart qi should go down to warm the feet, kidney qi should rise to moisten and cool the brain, calming and nourishing the spirit. In the interplay between these two qi, each keeps the other in balance. When fire is out of control, the best approach is to use water to bring it back into proper proportion. In this way the ruler is regulated and supported without being weakened. This may be accomplished by supplementing the kidneys with acupuncture points such as *Tai Xi* (Ki 3) or *San Yin Jiao* (Sp 6).

Appendix C

Examples of Other Point Formulas Involving
Zu San Li (St 36), *San Yin Jiao* (Sp 6), *He Gu* (LI 4),
Qu Chi (LI 11), & *Lie Que* (Lu 7)

Zu San Li (St 36)

Zu San Li (St 36) combined with *He Gu* (LI 4) regulates the middle and increases digestion. Stimulation of *Zu San Li* (St 36) increases peristalsis in the stomach, causing faster, stronger activity. Stimulation of *He Gu* (LI 4) however, makes the stomach's movements slower. The two used together resolve stomach spasm and spasm of the pyloric sphincter which causes vomiting. Because of the self-regulating action of these points *Zu San Li* (St 36) and *He Gu* (LI 4) together can decrease movement in the stomach if it is too fast and can increase it if it is too weak.

Zu San Li (St 36) can be used to stop pain and spasm anywhere in the body. In the upper burner it is used for headache, sore throat, tooth ache, and stiff neck, and any kind of tetany, for instance lock jaw and spasms experienced by paralysis patients. It helps facial prolapse and wry mouth after stroke and facial twitches. It can be used with *Ying Xiang* (LI 20) for any kind of sinus disease.

Zu San Li (St 36) increases lung capacity and brings down uprising qi. This makes it useful in the treatment of emphysema and empty or deficiency asthma. If the asthmatic attack is sudden and full or *shi*, drain *Zu San Li* (St 36). Because it relaxes the bronchi, its use tranquilizes and relaxes asthma patients. Difficulty breathing can be treated with *Zu San Li* (St 36), *He Gu* (LI 4), and *Lie Que* (Lu 7).

With *Lie Que* (Lu 7), it searches for wind and rids wetness and can be used for all bronchial problems. Together these points stop wheezing and transform phlegm, whether due to a full or an empty condition. If there is fullness, use *xie fa* or drainage. If there is emptiness, use *bu fa* or supplementation.

Zu San Li (St 36) helps to recede fever and clear heat by inducing perspiration. Use *Zu San Li* (St 36), *He Gu* (LI 4), and *Lie Que* (Lu 7) together for fever without perspiration. If there is already too much perspiration supplement *Fu Liu* (Ki 7) and drain *He Gu* (LI 4). In acute pneumonia *Zu San Li* (St 36), *He Gu* (LI 4), *Qu Chi* (LI 11), and *Da Zhu* (GV 14) increase the white blood cell count and fight infection. If, even after the disease is over, the person still has a low-grade fever, use *Zu San Li* (St 36), *He Gu* (LI 4), and *Qu Chi* (LI 11).

In the middle burner, in addition to regulating digestive activity, it is also used for chest, breast, and flank pain. It eliminates extravasated blood and so is used for traumatic injury and bruising of the chest. Bleed it for heart disease or drain Four Flower Middle.

In the lower burner, *Zu San Li* (St 36) treats intestinal pain and borborygmus, low back pain with ringing ear due to weak, empty kidneys, hip pain, swollen knees and foot pain. It balances the stomach and large intestine. Use it with *Zhi Gou* (TH 6) for constipation or with *Zhong Wan* (CV 12) for acute gastritis with simultaneous vomiting and diarrhea. *Zu San Li* (St 36), plus *He Gu* (LI 4) and *Qu Chi* (LI 11) stops diarrhea by increasing qi in the large intestine and lungs which are then able to hold up the stool against gravity. Ordinary loose stools or bowel movements soon after eating and indigestion which causes diarrhea in children can be helped by *Zu San Li* (St 36).

For gynecological problems, use *Zu San Li* (St 36), *San Yin Jiao* (Sp 6), *Zhi Gou* (TH 6) and *Qu Chi* (LI 11) to treat amenorrhea and post-partum dizziness. Acute menorrhagia can be treated with *Zu San Li* (St 36), *San Yin Jiao* (Sp 6), and *Zhong Ji* (CV 3).

Zu San Li (St 36) alone increases urination and dissolves swelling due to water retention. *San Yin Jiao* (Sp 6) can be added to treat edema. If water retention is more severe, add *He Gu* (LI 4) and *Qu Chi* (LI 11). *Zu San Li* (St 36) with *Yin Ling Quan* (Sp 9) treats difficult urination. If the abdomen is bloated due to water retention, first moxa *Shui Fen* (CV 9), and *Shui Dao* (St 28) which is 2 *cun* lateral to *Guan Yuan* (CV 4); then drain *Zu San Li* (St 36) and supplement *San Yin Jiao* (Sp 6).

Zu San Li (St 36), *San Yin Jiao* (Sp 6), and *Yang Ling Quan* (GB 34) are used for leg pain. *Zu San Li* should be stimulated for any difficulty walking both in children and adults and is especially indicated for paralysis due to polio. Use if for chronic knee pain due to arthritis or injury. If the knees are swollen round like balls, moxa *Zu San Li* (St 36).

For hypertension, use *Zu San Li* (St 36), *Nei Guan* (Per 6), and *San Yin Jiao* (Sp 6).

San Yin Jiao (Sp 6)

San Yin Jiao (Sp 6) is often used to treat digestive, urinary, and reproductive system problems. A few examples from the literature follow.

San Yin Jiao (Sp 6) and *Cheng Shan* (Bl 57) treat fullness in the lungs. *San Yin Jiao* (Sp 6) with *Zhong Wan* (CV 12), *Nei Guan* (Per 6), and *Zu San Li* (St 36) treat all conditions of bloated stomach, lower abdominal pain, and diarrhea. *San Yin Jiao* (Sp 6) plus *Nei Ting* (St 44) and *Zu San Li* (St 36) help all kinds of bloating.

For urogenital problems, *San Yin Jiao* (Sp 6) plus *Qi Hai* (CV 6) are indicated. Nocturnal emission in men and leukorrhea in women respond especially well to these 2 points. If there is enuresis or uncontrolled urination at night, use *San Yin Jiao* (Sp 6) and *Guan Yuan* (CV 4). If children experience urinary incontinence during the daytime, use *San Yin Jiao* (Sp 6), *Shen Shu* (Bl 23), *Pang Guang Shu* (Bl 28), and *Guan Yuan* (CV 4). These points can also be used for adults if there is no urination, for absence of erection in men due to kidney yang emptiness, and for menstrual pain in women.

Treat *San Yin Jiao* (Sp 6) and bleed *Wei Zhong* (Bl 40) for gonorrhea and pain of the penis. If the penis shrinks back into the body, becoming smaller, use *San Yin Jiao* (Sp 6) and *Tai Chong* (Liv 3). *San Yin Jiao* (Sp 6), *Da Dun* (Liv 1), and *Zu San Li* (St 36) can be used for any kind of hernia, especially of the testicles in which one is large and one is small. *San Yin Jiao* (Sp 6) and *Xue Hai* (Sp 10), *Guan Yuan* (CV 4) and *Qi Hai* (CV 6) treat irregular periods. For dreams of having sex leading to nocturnal emission for men and orgasm for women, supplement *San Yin Jiao* (Sp 6) and *Fu Liu* (Ki 7).

He Gu (LI 4)

Use right *He Gu* (LI 4) to treat left sided toothache and vice versa. If pain is in the lower jaw, use *He Gu* (LI 4) alone. If the upper jaw is in pain, combine it with *Zu San Li* (St 36) or *Nei Ting* (St 44).

Because of the large intestine's relationship with the lungs, *He Gu* (LI 4) and *Qu Chi* (LI 11) are always used to treat skin diseases, including boils, acne, and eczema. *He Gu* (LI 4) is also used for cough and asthma.

Caution! Supplementation of *He Gu* (LI 4) and drainage of *San Yin Jiao* can cause miscarriage. However, supplementation of *San Yin Jiao* (Sp 6) and drainage of *He Gu* (LI 4) can increase the body's firm hold on the fetus, thus preventing miscarriage. Any practitioner attempting this treatment must be absolutely certain of their technique. *San Yin Jiao* (Sp 6) takes care of yin blood. Blood should be supplemented, not drained. The lungs are in charge of the qi. They should be drained, not supplemented, even in the case of emptiness. If *San Yin Jiao* (Sp 6) is drained and *He Gu* (LI 4) is supplemented, the blood will be weakened and the qi will be excessive. In this condition, the pregnancy cannot hold. When the blood is strong and the qi is weak, the pregnancy will hold.

Cases of amenorrhea or lack of menstruation and excessive menstruation or menorrhagia can both be treated by supplementing *San Yin Jiao* (Sp 6) and draining *He Gu* (LI 4).

Lie Que (Lu 7)

For cold headache, direct the needle toward *Tai Yuan* (Lu 9) or with the direction of the channel's flow to supplement and combine it with *He Gu* (LI 4) and *Wai Guan* (TH 5). Otherwise *Lie Que* (Lu 7) is directed against the flow of the channel for drainage.

If combined with *Zu San Li* (St 36), *Lie Que* (Lu 7) treats bronchial asthma and cold cough. In the event of chest injury and bruising, bleed *Lie Que* (Lu 7) to relieve the pain. It can also be used for tetany or stiff neck, arched back, and eyes staring straight ahead.

Qu Chi (LI 11)

Because *Qu Chi* (LI 11) scatters wind and relieves the surface, it is a major point for treating skin disease of the whole body. Used to stop itching and prevent infection, it is known as a special point for the treatment of boils and pimples. *Qu Chi* (LI 11) paired with *San Yin Jiao* (Sp 6) clears heat and wind and cleanses heat from the blood. Many skin diseases are due to blood heat or *xue re*.

Qu Chi (LI 11) tranquilizes the spirit, reduces blood pressure, improves sleep, and treats madness of the type involving violence and talking nonsense. It relieves any kind of pain: arthritis, beri-beri, low back pain, dysmenorrhea, etc. It also relives pain and swelling of lumps which appear in the lower abdomen during menstruation.

Qu Chi (LI 11) plus *He Gu* (LI 4) treat head, face, ears, eyes, nose, and mouth. They are especially useful for conjunctivitis and for lesions of the eyelid but not sties. This kind of lesion is often seen in alcoholics, whose eyelashes may drop off. *Qu Chi* (LI 11) and *He Gu* (LI 4) also treat lack of coordination in the hands or difficulty holding things. Use these 2 for dysentery and other acute conditions. However, for chronic loose stool, treat the spleen.

In Chinese medicine, high blood pressure is due to liver yang rising. Low blood pressure is related to liver yin emptiness. Both can lead to dizziness. According to the 24 hour Chinese clock's flow of qi, liver qi goes to the lungs and then to the large intestine. Therefore, the large intestine can treat liver disease since metal also controls wood. Use *Qu Chi* (LI 11) to adjust blood pressure and relieve dizziness of the head, not of the eyes.

Appendix D

Illustrations of Extra Points

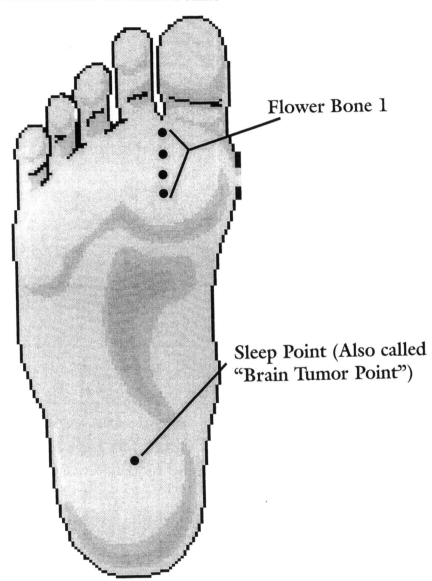

Flower Bone 1

Sleep Point (Also called "Brain Tumor Point")

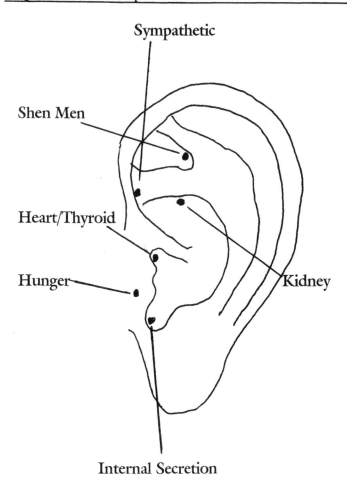

Sympathetic

Shen Men

Heart/Thyroid

Hunger

Kidney

Internal Secretion

Appendix E

Treatment of Acquired Immune Deficiency Syndrome or AIDS

In Chinese medicine, Acquired Immune Deficiency Syndrome, or AIDS, is considered to be a condition of severe depletion and malnutrition which results in the sufferer's inability to resist any disease, even the common cold. The healing process in AIDS is very slow, and lengthy moxa treatments, with the moxa burned in cans placed over the points rather than on needles, is the best approach. Needles are *not* avoided for fear of contagion. Because yin and yang are both empty and deficient and needling always causes some drainage, they are avoided to prevent further depletion. Moxa builds blood as well as qi, promotes the absorption of food, and enables the body to rebuild itself while providing qi to fight off disease.

Specific treatment depends on the individual's condition. Generally, we must first warm the stomach/middle burner to promote absorption. Below is outlined a typical course of treatment. These points increase the activity of the heart and regulate blood pressure as well as strengthening the middle.

Note that all points are treat with moxa, not needles.

Days 1   *Zhong Wan* (CV 12), *Zu San Li* (St 36), *Qi Hai* (CV 6), & 2 *Shen Que* (CV 8)
Day 3   *Xia Wan* (CV 10), *Tian Shu* (St 25), *Shen Que* (CV 8)
Day 4   *Huan Tiao* (GB 30), *Yang Ling Quan* (GB 34), *Shen Que* (CV 8)
Day 5   *Qi Men* (Liv 14), *Tai Chong* (Liv 3), *Shen Que* (CV 8)
Day 6   *Feng Shi* (GB 31), *Shen Mai* (Bl 62), *Shen Que* (CV 8)
Day 7   *Guan Yuan* (CV 4), *San Yin Jiao* (Sp 6), *Shen Que* (CV 8)
Day 8   *Jian Yu* (LI 15), *Qu Chi* (LI 11), *Shen Que* (CV 8)
Day 9   *Xin Shu* (Bl 15), *Shen Men* (Ht 7), *Shen Que* (CV 8)
Day 10   *Feng Chi* (GB 20), *Xuan Zhong* (GB 39), *Shen Que* (CV 8)
Day 11   *Ge Shu* (Bl 17), *Shan Zhong* (CV 17), *Ju Que* (CV 14), *Shen Que* (CV 8)
Day 12   *Shen Zhu* (GV 12), *Yao Yang Guan* (GV 3), *San Yin Jiao* (Sp 6), *Shen Que* (CV 8)

Day 13   *Jue Yin Shu* (Bl 14), *Shao Hai* (Ht 3), *Shen Que* (CV 8)
Day 14   *Wei Zhong* (Bl 40)*, *Zhao Hai* (Ki 6), *Shen Que* (CV 8)
Day 15   *Zhong Chong* (Per 1), *Jian Shi* (Per 5), *Shen Que* (CV 8)
Day 16   *Shen Shu* (Bl 23), *Zhao Hai* (Ki 6), *Shen Que* (CV 8)
Day 17   *Bai Hui* (GV 20)*, *Ya Men* (GV 15)*, *Lie Que* (Lu 7),
         Shen Que (CV 8)

* *Wei Zhong* (Bl 40) must be treated carefully to avoid blistering. Moxa at *Ya Men* (GV 15) is usually contraindicated. But in such severe situations, it is permitted. *Bai Hui* (GV 20) and *Ya Men* (GV 15) should not be given moxa too early, or headaches may occur. First clear congestion and open the passages using moxa on other points. This process usually takes 2 weeks of treatment. Then *Bai Hui* (GV 20) and *Ya Men* (GV 15) may be used. Each treatment lasts 30-40 minutes.

If no cans are available, use ginger and moxa for all points except *Ya Men* (GV 15) and *Wei Zhong* (Bl 40) which should be done with stick moxa.

If the patient catches a cold during the course of treatment, quickly moxa *Fei Shu* (Bl 12) and *Yang Ling Quan* (GB 34) until the cold is over or 3-4 days. If there is constipation, stop the regular treatment and moxa left *Da Heng* (Sp 15) and both *Cheng Shan* (Bl 57). Usually one treatment will cause the bowels to move, but it may be slower with AIDS patients.

Appendix F

Dietary Directions for Asthma/Emphysema Patients

In general avoid the following:
1. coldness outside the body, *i.e.,* exposure to chill and wind
2. cold foods and drinks
3. in severe cases, eat no raw foods
4. bathe with warm water only and avoid chill afterwards
5. reduce intake of sour foods, salt and salty foods
6. keep the chest warm and covered

Specifically do not have the following:
1. ice water/ice tea
2. wine
3. coffee or tea
4. soft drinks, especially colas
5. pineapple, banana, coconut (any part, even the oil as an ingredient)
6. bread or anything with yeast
7. curry, chilies, and other hot, spicy seasonings
8. Chinese cabbage (bok choy), winter melon, bamboo, bean sprouts, turnips
9. pickled vegetables (They are salty, which makes the phlegm stay in the lungs. The same applies to cheeses.)
10. tofu, unless deep fried or fried with green onions
11. salted fish
12. prawns, crab, or other shellfish
13. chicken, beef, mutton
14. raw eggs

For protein, pork is best, fish if cooked with ginger is good, hard boiled eggs, red or black beans.

Appendix G

Mental Degeneration — Stages of Progression Beginning With a Tight Stomach

Stage 1. Unhappiness, internal tension, nervousness. The person does not know what to do and is in conflict, but seems calm on the outside, saying little if anything about internal troubles. The stool is small, a sign of tenseness.

Stage 2. The mind runs in a circle. The patient mentally repeats what was said over and over. Urination increases, skin thickens and becomes wrinkled. There will be weight loss and dehydration. Appetite dwindles as does the ability to laugh and sleep. The patient hates fire and won't cook.

Stage 3. The patient cannot think, hates noise, especially the sound of tapping on wood (liver *vs.* kidneys). Such sounds produce shaking, depression, and fearfulness. If the heart is involved, they talk nonsense and will not listen, singing songs with no meaning at inappropriate times, laughing to himself, yelling in your office. People with such imbalances complain bitterly about the treatment you give them, scold, and threaten to sue. This is a full heart imbalance. Needle *Shen Men* (Ht 7) for a short time and do not take their insults and outrages personally. When the heart is empty, the patient will be unhappy, crying constantly. The pressures of adversity will seem unbearable. Again needle *Shen Men* (Ht 7) but leave the needle in longer.

Stage 4. At this stage, the patient has no shame. They may run naked through the streets, singing loudly and climbing trees, and may be suicidal or homicidal. This is due to too much stomach heat. Therefore, bleed *Li Dui* (St 45), the *jing* well point.

If the person loses sense of consciousness and the ability to talk, there is too much full heat and phlegm in the stomach. Drain *Feng Long* (St 40). If violent and raving, the person should be shut in a room for 2 days and made to drink their own urine. This causes him to vomit up phlegm, after which they will return to their senses.

Schizophrenic patients who repeat themselves and whose voices go from a whisper to a shout in the same sentence may not be getting enough blood to the brain. Use barefoot doctors' needles[7] down the spine and *Tong Li* (Ht 5).

At any stage, *Zu San Li* (St 36), *San Yin Jiao* (Sp 6), *He Gu* (LI 4), *Qu Chi* (LI 11), and *Lie Que* (Lu 7) will help calm the patient and restore balance to the internal organs so that the heart can again house the spirit.

---

[7] Barefoot doctors' needles is a description of a technique used traditionally in Northeastern China. In this method a relatively thick needle is inserted superficially and transversely along the Governing channel between the vertebrae. This method has been proven to have an analgesic, anti-allergic, and anti-inflammatory effect, helping to regulate the nervous and endocrine systems.

Appendix H

Winter Pear & Rock Sugar for Reducing Phlegm

These are the directions I give to patients with cough and excessive phlegm. I check for them the appropriate method of preparation and the best dosage.

Take 1 winter pear (the dark-skinned variety).
___Remove the skin if the phlegm is white.
___Do not remove the skin if phlegm is yellow.

Cut the pear in half, remove and discard the core. Fill the hole with approximately 1 tsp. rock sugar — break up sugar if necessary. Place pear with sugar in a pot, add 1 c. water.

Cover the pot with lid. Boil 15-20 minutes. Eat the pear and drink the liquid:
___at night upon retiring
___in the morning
___once a day
___twice a day

Explanation

Winter pear is cold as is rock sugar.[8] This coldness clears the spleen so that it will not produce too much phlegm. When boiled, the pear is medium cold. The skin is colder. Therefore, if phlegm is due to heat and is yellow, retain the skin. If the disease is deep, have the patient take this recipe twice a day. If they are not sleeping well, they should eat it before going to bed. If there is much phlegm in the morning, also take it then to facilitate expectoration.

---

8   While white sugar has little value and does the spleen much damage when consumed in excessive amounts, rock and brown sugar have medicinal properties and, in small amounts, they strengthen the spleen. That is why Chinese cough remedies contain sugar.

Appendix I

Not All Fever Is Caused by Infection

Case 1

A man, aged 69, had a kidney operation. For six weeks afterwards, his temperature was 99°F. His physician gave him antibiotics. One week later, his temperature averaged 100°F. The doctor increased the dosage of antibiotic. That week his temperature was 101°F. Again the doctor increased the antibiotics. After the third week, laboratory tests showed no infection, but still the fever remained and the patient became progressively worse.

The family called me to the house. The patient's pulse indicated weakness. Because of the antibiotics, he had no appetite. Because he could not eat, he could not recover. I looked into his eyes to tell him how serious his condition was and said, "If you believe my words, you will stop the antibiotics. Soak your feet in hot water twice a day, for 20 minutes each time."

I instructed his wife to buy a small game hen, steam it, and keep the broth. Then I went home and made egg noodles as thin as paper. The wife cooked the noodles in the broth and gave them to the man to eat. Beginning that afternoon at 4 PM, he soaked his feet 20 minutes and ate. At 9:45 that night, his fever was gone and did not return. From then on, he began to recover his strength.

Chinese medicine recognizes 2 kinds of fire or fever. Real or full fire is due to infection. Western laboratory tests find bacteria present. False or empty fire, which this patient had, is due to deficiency and extreme weakness. In this man's case, the stress of surgery depleted him even further after his illness. No bacteria are present, nor is there any infection. Rather, the body's qi is so depleted that an imbalance occurs in which the fire which normally goes down to warm the feet rises to the head and manifests as fever.

Soaking the feet in hot water serves to draw the empty fire down from the upper regions, sending it back to warm the feet. Proper nourishment must be provided at the same time to give the body enough strength to maintain the corrected balance. When dealing with this kind of yin empty fire, the patient should not sweat too much. The purpose of soaking in hot water is to bring down the heat, not to expel it through perspiration.

Whenever anyone is just beginning to catch cold and feels feverish, I tell them to soak their feet in hot water as soon as possible. They should cover themselves with a blanket and place their feet in hot running water, as hot as they can stand it, gradually increasing the temperature. The water level should not rise above the knee. Letting the hot water run until even the forehead and upper back perspire drives the heat out of the body. Even bacterial infection can be sweated out this way. Afterward, it is important to dry the head and chest and feet, go the bed, cover up with many blankets, and sleep. Because this condition is due to full, external evil, the treatment is stronger, aimed at getting rid of the heat.

Children under 3 years of age who wake crying and feverish in the night can be washed in hot but not too hot water from the legs to the buttocks, not the whole body, keeping the upper body well covered, warm and dry. All at once the child will stop crying and be able to sleep. It may still be advisable for them to have a treatment the next day, to be careful of what they eat, and to avoid getting chilled.

Case 2

A man, 63 years old, had angina and high cholesterol for 5 years. He had been treated by Western medicine, but the chest pains continued and he could no longer drive his car. He came for acupuncture which relieved the pain and he was able to drive again. When his grandson was born in Nevada, he wanted to go to see him. The place where his family lived was at a high altitude. I felt that the altitude and especially the plane ride would not be good for his heart, but he insisted on going. So I suggested that he stay for a short time only and get medication from his doctor in case the angina recurred. He stayed in Nevada for 4 days until the pain in his chest forced him to leave. When he returned, he also had a fever for which the doctor prescribed antibiotics.

When he came back to me for treatment, I was concerned about the side effects of the antibiotics. Because I saw that the fever was empty fire and was not due to an infection, I advised him to discontinue the antibiotics, but he was afraid to do so. Soon his lips were burned with internal heat. Inside his mouth, his tongue, and throat, all visible tissue was blistered. 2 days later, he was unable to pass urine or stool, his whole body ached, and he suffered intense abdominal pain. These were side effects of the antibiotic combined with the heart medication.

To my way of thinking, this was another case of empty fire. In the high altitude, he could not get the oxygen he was accustomed to, so his heart had to work faster than normal and the extra load on his heart produced heat. He thought I was joking when I told him to soak his feet in hot water. A week later, he died in the hospital.

Note on antibiotics: If there is no other medication to complicate the issue by producing heat, and the patient experiences digestive problems due to the antibiotics, give moxa on *Zu San Li* (St 36), *Zhong Wan* (CV 12), *San Yin Jiao* (Sp 6), and *Qu Chi* (LI 11). Can moxa may be used on *Guan Yuan* (CV 4) as well.

Index

CONTROLLING DIABETES NATURALLY WITH
CHINESE MEDICINE
by Lynn Kuchinski
ISBN 0-936185-06-3
ISBN 978-0-936185-06-2

CURING ARTHRITIS NATURALLY WITH
CHINESE MEDICINE
by Douglas Frank & Bob Flaws
ISBN 0-936185-87-2
ISBN 978-0-936185-87-3

CURING DEPRESSION NATURALLY WITH
CHINESE MEDICINE
by Rosa Schnyer & Bob Flaws
ISBN 0-936185-94-5
ISBN 978-0-936185-94-1

CURING FIBROMYALGIA NATURALLY WITH
CHINESE MEDICINE
by Bob Flaws
ISBN 1-891845-09-8
ISBN 978-1-891845-09-3

CURING HAY FEVER NATURALLY WITH
CHINESE MEDICINE
by Bob Flaws
ISBN 0-936185-91-0
ISBN 978-0-936185-91-0

CURING HEADACHES NATURALLY WITH
CHINESE MEDICINE
by Bob Flaws
ISBN 0-936185-95-3
ISBN 978-0-936185-95-8

CURING IBS NATURALLY WITH CHINESE
MEDICINE
by Jane Bean Oberski
ISBN 1-891845-11-X
ISBN 978-1-891845-11-6

CURING INSOMNIA NATURALLY WITH
CHINESE MEDICINE
by Bob Flaws
ISBN 0-936185-86-4
ISBN 978-0-936185-86-6

CURING PMS NATURALLY WITH CHINESE
MEDICINE
by Bob Flaws
ISBN 0-936185-85-6
ISBN 978-0-936185-85-9

DISEASES OF THE KIDNEY & BLADDER
by Hoy Ping Yee Chan, et al.
ISBN 1-891845-37-3
ISBN 978-1-891845-35-6

THE DIVINE FARMER'S MATERIA MEDICA
A Translation of the Shen Nong Ben Cao
translation by Yang Shouz-zhong
ISBN 0-936185-96-1
ISBN 978-0-936185-96-5

DUI YAO: THE ART OF COMBINING
CHINESE HERBAL MEDICINALS
by Philippe Sionneau
ISBN 0-936185-81-3
ISBN 978-0-936185-81-1

ENDOMETRIOSIS, INFERTILITY AND
TRADITIONAL CHINESE MEDICINE:
A Layperson's Guide
by Bob Flaws
ISBN 0-936185-14-7
ISBN 978-0-936185-14-9

THE ESSENCE OF LIU FENG-WU'S GYNECOLOGY
by Liu Feng-wu, translated by Yang Shou-zhong
ISBN 0-936185-88-0
ISBN 978-0-936185-88-0

EXTRA TREATISES BASED ON INVESTIGATION &
INQUIRY: A Translation of Zhu Dan-xi's Ge Zhi Yu
Lun
translation by Yang Shou-zhong
ISBN 0-936185-53-8
ISBN 978-0-936185-53-8

FIRE IN THE VALLEY: TCM Diagnosis & Treatment of
Vaginal Diseases
by Bob Flaws
ISBN 0-936185-25-2
ISBN 978-0-936185-25-5

FULFILLING THE ESSENCE:
A Handbook of Traditional & Contemporary
Treatments for Female Infertility
by Bob Flaws
ISBN 0-936185-48-1
ISBN 978-0-936185-48-4

FU QING-ZHU'S GYNECOLOGY
trans. by Yang Shou-zhong and Liu Da-wei
ISBN 0-936185-35-X
ISBN 978-0-936185-35-4

GOLDEN NEEDLE WANG LE-TING: A 20th Century
Master's Approach to Acupuncture
by Yu Hui-chan and Han Fu-ru, trans. by Shuai Xue-zhong
ISBN 0-936185-78-3
ISBN 978-0-936185-78-1

A HANDBOOK OF CHINESE HEMATOLOGY
by Simon Becker
ISBN 1-891845-16-0
ISBN 978-1-891845-16-1

A HANDBOOK OF TCM PATTERNS
& THEIR TREATMENTS   Second Edition
by Bob Flaws & Daniel Finney
ISBN 0-936185-70-8
ISBN 978-0-936185-70-5

A HANDBOOK OF TRADITIONAL
CHINESE DERMATOLOGY
 by Liang Jian-hui, trans. by Zhang Ting-liang
& Bob Flaws
ISBN 0-936185-46-5
ISBN 978-0-936185-46-0

A HANDBOOK OF TRADITIONAL
CHINESE GYNECOLOGY
by Zhejiang College of TCM, trans. by Zhang Ting-liang
& Bob Flaws
ISBN 0-936185-06-6 (4th edit.)
ISBN 978-0-936185-06-4

A HANDBOOK of TCM PEDIATRICS
by Bob Flaws
ISBN 0-936185-72-4
ISBN 978-0-936185-72-9

THE HEART & ESSENCE OF DAN-XI'S
METHODS OF TREATMENT
by Xu Dan-xi, trans. by Yang Shou-zhong
ISBN 0-926185-50-3
ISBN 978-0-936185-50-7

HERB TOXICITIES & DRUG INTERACTIONS:
A Formula Approach
by Fred Jennes with Bob Flaws
ISBN 1-891845-26-8
ISBN 978-1-891845-26-0

IMPERIAL SECRETS OF HEALTH & LONGEVITY
by Bob Flaws
ISBN 0-936185-51-1
ISBN 978-0-936185-51-4

INSIGHTS OF A SENIOR ACUPUNCTURIST
by Miriam Lee
ISBN 0-936185-33-3
ISBN 978-0-936185-33-0

INTEGRATED PHARMACOLOGY: Combining Modern
Pharmacology with Chinese Medicine
by Dr. Greg Sperber with Bob Flaws
ISBN 1-891845-41-1
ISBN 978-0-936185-41-3

INTRODUCTION TO THE USE OF
PROCESSED CHINESE MEDICINALS
by Philippe Sionneau
ISBN 0-936185-62-7
ISBN 978-0-936185-62-0

KEEPING YOUR CHILD HEALTHY WITH
CHINESE MEDICINE
by Bob Flaws
ISBN 0-936185-71-6
ISBN 978-0-936185-71-2

THE LAKESIDE MASTER'S STUDY OF THE PULSE
by Li Shi-zhen, trans. by Bob Flaws
ISBN 1-891845-01-2
ISBN 978-1-891845-01-7

MANAGING MENOPAUSE NATURALLY WITH
CHINESE MEDICINE
by Honora Lee Wolfe
ISBN 0-936185-98-8
ISBN 978-0-936185-98-9

MASTER HUA'S CLASSIC OF THE CENTRAL
VISCERA
by Hua Tuo, trans. by Yang Shou-zhong
ISBN 0-936185-43-0
ISBN 978-0-936185-43-9

THE MEDICAL I CHING: Oracle of the Healer Within
by Miki Shima
ISBN 0-936185-38-4
ISBN 978-0-936185-38-5

MENOPAIUSE & CHINESE MEDICINE
by Bob Flaws
ISBN 1-891845-40-3
ISBN 978-1-891845-40-6

MOXIBUSTION: A MODERN CLINICAL HANDBOOK
by Lorraine Wilcox
ISBN 1-891845-49-7
ISBN 978-1-891845-49-9

MOXIBUSTION: THE POWER OF MUGWORT FIRE
by Lorraine Wilcox
ISBN 1-891845-46-2
ISBN 978-1-891845-46-8

A NEW AMERICAN ACUPUNTURE By Mark Seem
ISBN 0-936185-44-9
ISBN 978-0-936185-44-6

PLAYING THE GAME: A Step-by-Step Approach to
Accepting Insurance as an Acupuncturist
by Greg Sperber & Tiffany Anderson-Hefner
ISBN 3-131416-11-7
ISBN 978-3-131416-11-7

POCKET ATLAS OF CHINESE MEDICINE
Edited by Marne and Kevin Ergil
ISBN 1-891-845-59-4
ISBN 978-1-891845-59-8

POINTS FOR PROFIT: The Essential Guide to Practice
Success for Acupuncturists 4rd Edition
by Honora Wolfe, Eric Strand & Marilyn Allen
ISBN 1-891845-25-X
ISBN 978-1-891845-25-3

PRINCIPLES OF CHINESE MEDICAL ANDROLOGY:
An Integrated Approach to Male Reproductive and
Urological Health by Bob Damone
ISBN 1-891845-45-4
ISBN 978-1-891845-45-1

PRINCE WEN HUI's COOK: Chinese Dietary Therapy
By Bob Flaws & Honora Wolfe
ISBN 0-912111-05-4
ISBN 978-0-912111-05-6

THE PULSE CLASSIC:
A Translation of the Mai Jing
by Wang Shu-he, trans. by Yang Shou-zhong
ISBN 0-936185-75-9
ISBN 978-0-936185-75-0

THE SECRET OF CHINESE PULSE DIAGNOSIS
by Bob Flaws
ISBN 0-936185-67-8
ISBN 978-0-936185-67-5

SECRET SHAOLIN FORMULAS FOR THE
TREATMENT OF EXTERNAL INJURY
by De Chan, trans. by Zhang Ting-liang & Bob Flaws
ISBN 0-936185-08-2
ISBN 978-0-936185-08-8

STATEMENTS OF FACT IN TRADITIONAL
CHINESE MEDICINE   Revised & Expanded
by Bob Flaws
ISBN 0-936185-52-X
ISBN 978-0-936185-52-1

STICKING TO THE POINT: A Step-by-Step Approach
to TCM Acupuncture Therapy
by Bob Flaws & Honora Wolfe   2 Condensed Books
ISBN 1-891845-47-0
ISBN 978-1-891845-47-5

A STUDY OF DAOIST ACUPUNCTURE
by Liu Zheng-cai
ISBN 1-891845-08-X
ISBN 978-1-891845-08-6

THE SUCCESSFUL CHINESE HERBALIST
by Bob Flaws and Honora Lee Wolfe
ISBN 1-891845-29-2
ISBN 978-1-891845-29-1

THE SYSTEMATIC CLASSIC OF ACUPUNCTURE &
MOXIBUSTION
A translation of the Jia Yi Jing
by Huang-fu Mi, trans. by Yang Shou-zhong & Charles Chace
ISBN 0-936185-29-5
ISBN 978-0-936185-29-3

THE TAO OF HEALTHY EATING: DIETARY
WISDOM ACCORDING TO CHINESE MEDICINE
by Bob Flaws   Second Edition
ISBN 0-936185-92-9
ISBN 978-0-936185-92-7

TEACH YOURSELF TO READ MODERN
MEDICAL CHINESE
by Bob Flaws
ISBN 0-936185-99-6
ISBN 978-0-936185-99-6

TEST PREP WORKBOOK FOR BASIC TCM THEORY
by Zhong Bai-song
ISBN 1-891845-43-8
ISBN 978-1-891845-43-7

TEST PREP WORKBOOK FOR THE NCCAOM BIO-
MEDICINE MODULE: Exam Preparation & Study Guide
by Zhong Bai-song
ISBN 1-891845-34-9
ISBN 978-1-891845-34-5

TREATING PEDIATRIC BED-WETTING WITH
ACUPUNCTURE & CHINESE MEDICINE
by Robert Helmer
ISBN 1-891845-33-0
ISBN 978-1-891845-33-8

TREATISE on the SPLEEN & STOMACH: A
Translation and annotation of Li Dong-yuan's
Pi Wei Lun
by Bob Flaws
ISBN 0-936185-41-4
ISBN 978-0-936185-41-5

THE TREATMENT OF CARDIOVASCULAR DIS-
EASES WITH CHINESE MEDICINE
by Simon Becker, Bob Flaws &
Robert Casañas, MD
ISBN 1-891845-27-6
ISBN 978-1-891845-27-7

THE TREATMENT OF DIABETES MELLITUS WITH
CHINESE MEDICINE
by Bob Flaws, Lynn Kuchinski &
Robert Casañas, M.D.
ISBN 1-891845-21-7
ISBN 978-1-891845-21-5

THE TREATMENT OF DISEASE IN TCM, Vol. 1:
Diseases of the Head & Face, Including Mental &
Emotional Disorders   New Edition
by Philippe Sionneau & Lü Gang
ISBN 0-936185-69-4
ISBN 978-0-936185-69-9

THE TREATMENT OF DISEASE IN TCM, Vol. II:
Diseases of the Eyes, Ears, Nose, & Throat
by Sionneau & Lü
ISBN 0-936185-73-2
ISBN 978-0-936185-73-6

THE TREATMENT OF DISEASE IN TCM, Vol. III:
Diseases of the Mouth, Lips, Tongue, Teeth & Gums
by Sionneau & Lü
ISBN 0-936185-79-1
ISBN 978-0-936185-79-8

THE TREATMENT OF DISEASE IN TCM, Vol IV:
Diseases of the Neck, Shoulders, Back, & Limbs
by Philippe Sionneau & Lü Gang
ISBN 0-936185-89-9
ISBN 978-0-936185-89-7

THE TREATMENT OF DISEASE IN TCM, Vol V:
Diseases of the Chest & Abdomen
by Philippe Sionneau & Lü Gang
ISBN 1-891845-02-0
ISBN 978-1-891845-02-4

THE TREATMENT OF DISEASE IN TCM, Vol VI:
Diseases of the Urogential System & Proctology
by Philippe Sionneau & Lü Gang
ISBN 1-891845-05-5
ISBN 978-1-891845-05-5

THE TREATMENT OF DISEASE IN TCM, Vol VII:
General Symptoms
by Philippe Sionneau & Lü Gang
ISBN 1-891845-14-4
ISBN 978-1-891845-14-7

THE TREATMENT OF EXTERNAL DISEASES WITH
ACUPUNCTURE & MOXIBUSTION
by Yan Cui-lan and Zhu Yun-long, trans. by Yang Shou-zhong
ISBN 0-936185-80-5
ISBN 978-0-936185-80-4

THE TREATMENT OF MODERN WESTERN
MEDICAL DISEASES WITH CHINESE MEDICINE
by Bob Flaws & Philippe Sionneau
ISBN 1-891845-20-9
ISBN 978-1-891845-20-8

UNDERSTANDING THE DIFFICULT PATIENT: A
Guide for Practitioners of Oriental Medicine
by Nancy Bilello, RN, L.ac.
ISBN 1-891845-32-2
ISBN 978-1-891845-32-1

WESTERN PHYSICAL EXAM SKILLS FOR
PRACTITIONERS OF ASIAN MEDICINE
by Bruce H. Robinson & Honora Lee Wolfe
ISBN 1-891845-48-9
ISBN 978-1-891845-48-2

YI LIN GAI CUO (Correcting the Errors in the Forest of
Medicine)
by Wang Qing-ren
ISBN 1-891845-39-X
ISBN 978-1-891845-39-0

70 ESSENTIAL CHINESE HERBAL FORMULAS
by Bob Flaws
ISBN 0-936185-59-7
ISBN 978-0-936185-59-0

160 ESSENTIAL CHINESE READY-MADE
MEDICINES
by Bob Flaws
ISBN 1-891945-12-8
ISBN 978-1-891945-12-3

630 QUESTIONS & ANSWERS ABOUT CHINESE
HERBAL MEDICINE:
A Workbook & Study Guide
by Bob Flaws
ISBN 1-891845-04-7
ISBN 978-1-891845-04-8

260 ESSENTIAL CHINESE MEDICINALS
by Bob Flaws
ISBN 1-891845-03-9
ISBN 978-1-891845-03-1

750 QUESTIONS & ANSWERS ABOUT
ACUPUNCTURE
Exam Preparation & Study Guide
by Fred Jennes
ISBN 1-891845-22-5
ISBN 978-1-891845-22-2